Reiki Healing For Beginners

Awaken Your Chakras and Increase Self-healing

(Awaken Your Spiritual Power, Reduce Stress & Anxiety and Improve Awareness of Psychic Abilities)

Tanmaya McKenzie

Published by Rob Miles

Tanmaya McKenzie

All Rights Reserved

Reiki Healing for Beginners: Awaken Your Chakras and Increase Self-healing (Awaken Your Spiritual Power, Reduce Stress & Anxiety and Improve Awareness of Psychic Abilities)

ISBN 978-1-989990-28-5

All rights reserved. No part of this guide may be reproduced in any form without permission in writing from the publisher except in the case of brief quotations embodied in critical articles or reviews.

Legal & Disclaimer

The information contained in this book is not designed to replace or take the place of any form of medicine or professional medical advice. The information in this book has been provided for educational and entertainment purposes only.

The information contained in this book has been compiled from sources deemed reliable, and it is accurate to the best of the Author's knowledge; however, the Author cannot guarantee its accuracy and validity and cannot be held liable for any errors or omissions. Changes are periodically made to this book. You must consult your doctor or get professional medical advice before using any of the suggested remedies, techniques, or information in this book.

Upon using the information contained in this book, you agree to hold harmless the Author from and against any damages, costs, and expenses, including any legal fees potentially resulting from the application of any of the information provided by this guide. This disclaimer applies to any damages or injury caused by the use and application, whether directly or indirectly, of any advice or information presented, whether for breach of contract, tort, negligence, personal injury, criminal intent, or under any other cause of action.

You agree to accept all risks of using the information presented inside this book. You need to consult a professional medical practitioner in order to ensure you are both able and healthy enough to participate in this program.

Table of Contents

INTRODUCTION 1

CHAPTER 1: BENEFITS OF REIKI HEALING 3

CHAPTER 2: REIKI SYMBOLS AND MEANINGS 9

CHAPTER 3: WHAT IS REIKI? BASIC FACTS YOU SHOULD KNOW 24

CHAPTER 4: WHAT YOU SHOULD KNOW ABOUT REIKI AS A BEGINNER 40

CHAPTER 5: REIKI SYMBOLS AND THEIR UNIQUE USES 60

CHAPTER 6: TIME FOR CHANGE 69

CHAPTER 7: HEAL YOURSELF 82

CHAPTER 8: BENEFITS OF REIKI 98

CHAPTER 9: HOW REIKI CAN HELP REDUCE STRESS 118

CHAPTER 10: INCREASE YOUR ENERGY WITH REIKI 125

CHAPTER 11: THE SIGNS 130

CHAPTER 12: SYMBOLS OF REIKI 149

CHAPTER 13: REIKI SECTION 164

CHAPTER 14: HARNESSING THE POWER OF REIKI 175

CHAPTER 15: REIKI HEALING SUCCESS SORIES **183**

CHAPTER 16: REIKI AND AROMATHERAPY **189**

CONCLUSION **195**

Introduction

Reiki is a spiritual practice everybody can learn from a qualified teacher. Learning what is commonly referred to as Japanese Reiki is simple, but it requires time like most good things in life. It also needs the ability to acquire, based on your awareness. A person cannot receive more than the level he can reach, determined by the standard he resonates with. This may sound not very easy, but it's not with a Reiki Shihan.

Furthermore, Reiki is a powerful cure device that allows a practitioner to place his or her hands on the customer without really controlling the body. It makes Reiki an excellent healing method for people suffering from physical and emotional problems of all kinds. Most clinics now provide Reiki healing as a relief and quicker treatment for their patients.

Also, this offers specific methods for achieving and sustaining internal peace and happiness, power, and immune systems. Methods include techniques of mindfulness and imagination, reflection, and meaningful thinking.

Conclusively, Reiki also provides a potent cure for any emotional "baggage," whether it's sorrow, anger, sadness or fear by smoothly releasing such emotions, usually without major disaster or curves. Reiki operates through the very gentle liberation of suppressed feelings just by harmonizing the negative impact and allowing energy to be released or recycled by the body.

Chapter 1: Benefits Of Reiki Healing

Although Reiki treatments are simple, it produces profound healing effects on our body and mind. Reiki therapy is not only to heal and improve the quality of your physical body but also the mind and the spirit resulting in increased joy in your life. The best thing about Reiki treatment is that it is not only for sick people. Even the healthy ones can experience increased joy and happiness through Reiki healing practices. Let us look at some of the fabulous benefits of Reiki:

It promotes balance and harmony – Reiki works at restoring your natural energy levels while promoting overall wellness. It works at the roots of problems and solves them instead of finding only symptomatic relief or merely masking symptoms. Creating balance and harmony happens at various levels between different pairs of opposing elements including:

- Emotional and mental
- Left and right sides of the brain
- Feminine and masculine attributes
- Labeling elements and things as good or bad
- Negative and positive aspects of your life

It creates relaxation and stress-relief at a very deep level – During Reiki treatments, you are just 'being' and not 'doing' anything. Nearly every practitioner feels a sense of calm, peace, clarity, and relaxation after Reiki sessions. Reiki sessions allow you to become increasingly self-aware of your body sensations and feelings resulting in being 'in the moment.' Being mindfully present in the moment enhances your life experiences and helps you relax and de-stress.

It dissolves energy blocks in your system and facilitates self-healing – Reiki can heal physical and mental wounds by removing and clearing off energy blocks in your system. It can help clear off negative emotions such as anger, fear, resentment, jealousy, etc. Reiki improves your ability to love resulting in attracting more people in your life than before.

Reiki treatments are designed to return your body to its naturally balanced state. This means your breathing rate, your heart rate, and blood pressure are all restored to their natural levels of normalcy. In fact, Reiki sessions help in breathing easier and more deeply than before. Improved breathing is a critical element needed for increased self-healing tendencies of our body and mind.

It cleanses and removes toxins from your system – Our modern life is so stressed out that we are constantly in a flight-fight mode resulting in overuse of our sympathetic nervous system. This situation, in turn, results in excessive release of stress hormones in our body, which accumulate as toxins in our body. As a result, in being in a flight/fight mode, you will be exhausted, tired, and drained of energy at all times.

Reiki treatments remind our bodies to use the parasympathetic nervous system also referred to as rest and digest system resulting in self-healing mode. As you practice Reiki regularly, your body will be habituated to using the parasympathetic system resulting in the reduction and release of toxins from your body. Moreover, the increased use of the parasympathetic nervous system thereby results in improved energy levels without feeling exhausted and burned out.

It improves sleep – The relaxation associated with Reiki sessions result in restful sleep at night. A good night's rest has multiple benefits including improved healing of your body and mind, increased clarity of thought, and more.

Reiki heals physical body problems too – While Reiki treatments appear to be something as simple as 'placing hands' on the various parts of the body, it is so powerful that it restores your body and mind at the deepest level. Reiki drives your body to improve its vital functioning so that your body is working at its optimal efficiency.

Moreover, Reiki therapy is known to alleviate pains of migraines, sciatica, arthritis, menopausal symptoms, and more. It is also known to cure chronic fatigue, asthma, and insomnia.

Reiki helps emotional cleansing and spiritual growth – As Reiki addresses your entire being instead of only focusing on one aspect, it facilitates emotional cleansing and spiritual growth as well. It can create subtle energy shifts in the deepest parts of your mind and spirit and alter your perceptions and outlook on life.

It can bring about positive changes in your attitude, an increased belief in your life purpose, and the reason for your being here at this point in time. You can perceive your situation in a new light empowering you to solve problems that hitherto seemed irresolvable. An inner shift in your belief system and spiritual energy can lead you to live a more spiritually-inspired life than before.

Considering the multiple benefits Reiki has to offer, it would be naïve not to learn and take advantage of this non-invasive, simple, and side-effects-free system of healing. And finally, Reiki can be learned and practiced on yourself. You don't need to go in hunt of a Reiki healer once you have mastered the skills.

Chapter 2: Reiki Symbols And Meanings

Reiki refers to a powerful medium that makes use of various symbols to promote healing. The symbols allow Reiki practitioners to heal other people effectively.

The various Reiki symbols form a high level of spirituality, awareness, and exhaling; they are a result of the Sanskrit language, which is understood to be a language of the spirits. Each symbol comes with a specific meaning that you can use to boost up your energy.

They can be used for protection and effective healing of the body and the mind. Let us look at the various symbols and their meanings.

Cho Ku Rei

Every Reiki session starts with this symbol because it forms the source of the energy that you will use in the session. The symbol means that all the power of the universe is taken and brought here.

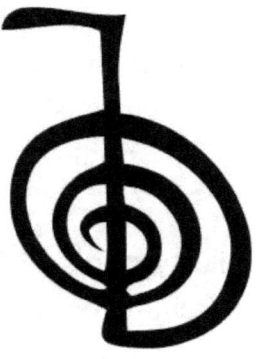

This symbol will enhance all the other powers of the symbols that you will use for that session. Using the symbol, you have the capacity to ad power to the various tools that you will use, such as the machines, medicines and other tools that you will utilize.

This symbol also eliminates the inflow of negative energy into the healing session.

This symbol can be used to cleanse the room of any negative energy that is in the room. Remember that the symbol itself doesn't give you the power that you need, but it acts as the connection to the power that you will use in the session.

The Cho Ku Rei acts as a connection to various sources of Reiki energy. You can draw this symbol in various ways, but the good thing is that they are all effective when used the right way.

Once you have an idea of the various symbols, you will have to use them at the conscious and subconscious levels for life. Rather than look at the various variations that each symbol comes with, it is better to look at what the symbol can do for you.

This symbol is usually called the "light switch" because it is seen as the one that brings to life all the other symbols. The three words in the symbol all have some meaning:

CHO – this is all about removing any illusion with the aim of connecting to the truth.

KU – Penetration of the truth so that you can get to the deepest level.

REI – a universal form of truth that is present everywhere.

Nearly all of the Reiki practitioners start every treatment by activating this symbol. By doing so, the practitioner starts the process that will turn on the switch, which will activate any healing powers that are needed to make things work.

You can draw the symbol in a clockwise or an anticlockwise direction. Regardless of the way you draw it, the intention is all that matters.

Uses

· This symbol activates the session to use the 2nd degree of Reiki energy.

· It activate all the other symbols to make them active.

· It also offers protection from all the levels.

· It cleanses energies in the home, car, and office.

· It balances your life.

· You can send the energy along with a sticker.

· It can be used on plants, food, and animals.

· It can be used to grow your career. You can draw the symbols under your cash register, desk, and telephone diary.

You can use the energy on whatever you desire to add positive energy to. These can be things or people.

Sei He ki

This symbol seems to have two meanings. The first meaning is all about trying to get a connection to your emotions, and the second one is all about you and God becoming one.

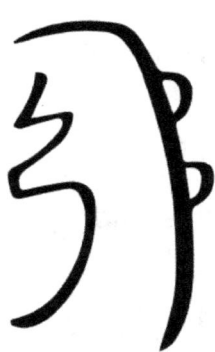

The symbol is aimed at trying to get you to acknowledge your emotions and feelings in such a way that you become one with the emotions. The symbol is ideal for understanding your emotional needs and then to deal with any issues that are associated with it.

Due to this, the symbol is able to handle any negative energy that is surrounding you and then helps to balance the emotions so that you can be a better person.

It is ideal for use against emotional trauma, jealousy, and frustration.

This symbol brings together the body and the brain and will help you to bring to the surface any emotional and mental issues that surround them.

Many practitioners and individuals start realizing that many of their problems are associated with mental imbalances that we aren't even aware of. The use of the symbols will help focus on the subconscious as well as the physical side.

The symbol is ideal for the mental and emotional healing that you can use. It helps give you harmony and peace.

Uses

· It can be utilized to help heal the misuse of alcohol, drugs, and smoking.

· Can help you lose weight.

· Can help you locate something that you have misplaced.

· Help in the healing process.

- You can use the symbol by drawing it in mid-air towards the direction that you wish the energy to go.

- Use the tongue to draw the symbol on top of your mouth then project it on top of your hands to use them on the client.

- Visualize the symbol to be strong on your palms before you can use them on the client.

- You can also do the same on the back of hands so that you can use them on the client.

- Draw the symbol on the palms using the index finger before you place them on a client.

For you to activate the second symbol, you need to use a method called the Reiki sandwich. You need first to draw and then activate Cho Ku rei symbol. Then go ahead and draw the Sei Hei Ki symbol and then activate it after which you draw the power symbol on it. This will help release the energy then allow the healing process to start.

Hon Sha Ze Sho Nen (Distance Healing Symbol)

It can be used to transfer energy over a certain distance. When a practitioner uses the Reiki symbols, time, and distance don't matter at all. Many practitioners consider this symbol to be the best ever, and it helps give access to life records that will help heal the body and the mind.

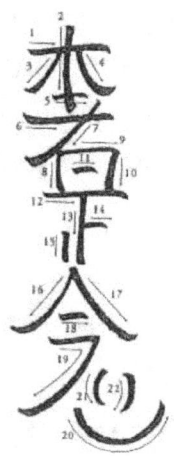

The symbol helps to handle traumatic and other experiences of life that affect other people, and that can be brought to the surface and get released.

When you decide to do long-distance healing, try and be open. Many people focus on trying to heal a specific part of the body, such as the headache or the feet. Instead, send out the Reiki energy without any limitation so that the energy will work on the whole body.

The good thing is that when you send out the Reiki energy, the other person will likely see things happening and will feel it. You can even use this symbol to send repeat energies to the person who needs the healing

Uses

· You can send Reiki healing to a person that is far from you.

· You can beam the Reiki energies to someone that is across the room or in another room.

· Send the energy to the future to help with a specific task or to work as support.

· Send the energy to the past so that you can lift up, release and understand.

Dai Ko Myo

This seems to be the most powerful symbol of all the rest, and it shows that every person has something unique to offer. The symbol helps to establish a very strong connection to your spirit as well as your higher self.

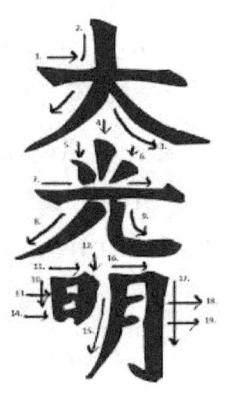

When you use the symbol, you get to nurture yourself as well as the people that are around you.

This symbol adds some momentum to the session and helps take the session to a whole different level.

This symbol cannot be used by just anyone but only the masters of Reiki. The power of this symbol is due to it combining all the other three symbols. It is the symbol that has the highest level of vibrations and therefore is the most transformative of all.

When you use the symbol, you enhance the healing of your soul since the energies are sent to all the layers of the mind.

The aim of the symbol is in such a way that when the soul gets healed, then the mental, as well as the physical issues, also get healed.

When the Reiki practitioner gets connected to the Reiki symbol by the master, the symbol will enter into its own chakra, and it will enlighten you about you really are. The symbol also helps you to associate your divinity with everything.

The symbol connects you to the divinity that you inherit and helps to heal yourself and others. This allows the energy to get an extra boost and then helps you to draw energy to your system.

Uses

· You can use the Reiki master to open the various channels during healing.

· Helps enhance the connection between one person to another and the universal energy that helps to heal the soul.

· Help deal with the diseases that come from conscious beliefs.

· Provide enlightenment.

· Helps you to develop and strengthen self-awareness, personal growth, and spiritual development.

· It helps increase the effectiveness of all other symbols to make them more effective.

- Used to charge crystals to make them heal better.
- Can be used to energize the immunity.
- Can be applied to herb tinctures and other remedies to make them stronger.

How to Use the Reiki Symbols to Develop a Positive Mindset

Let us look at the different ways you can apply the Reiki symbols to developing a positive mindset.

If you have ever run out of steam just because you have been in a wrong relationship or you have been in a situation, you need to find a way to release the energy. Let us look at the various ways you can manage your emotions.

It is ideal that you take baby steps to try and ease out the negative thought patterns that plague you.

1. Cho Ku Rei

When you wish to get out of the loop and be someone better, you need first to have an intention. This symbol will give you power over the universe so that you can direct your thoughts to something useful. This power symbol helps you to release any resistance. You can then set an intention to get out of any particular income.

2. Sei He Ki

When you focus on this symbol, you will have to bring balance in your life. Once you have detached yourself from the issue, you will have to proceed to mental and emotional healing. Say the symbol out loud so that you shift your attention towards mental healing.

If you are looking to memorize new information or ace your test, this symbol can help you do this. You can use the symbol on a book so that you get to memorize the information not just for a few hours but days and weeks.

3. Hon Sha Ze Sho Nen

This symbol helps you to go past time and space. You can use this energy to handle past unresolved issues or even handle issues that happened in a past life. You can also channel the energy to future situations such as interviews and meetings.

Chapter 3: What Is Reiki? Basic Facts You Should Know

Reiki is a treatment which is popularly known as hands healing in which a professional puts hands softly on or over a patient's body to encourage the patient's process of recuperating.

The word 'Reiki' is a combination of Japanese and Chinese word-characters.

Rei -- Profound or Powerful

Ki – imperative vitality

The basic idea shared by the individuals who practice Reiki is that this indispensable vitality can be directed to help the body's natural capacity to mend itself, as indicated by the National Center for Complementary and Integrative Health (NCCIH).

As indicated by these specialists, energy will be low in the body where there has been physical damage or conceivably emotional instability. Sickness itself is a result of these energy reductions.

Energy healing is centered at progressing the flow of vitality and eliminate blocks; this is also done in acupuncture and acupressure. Researchers believe that improving the progression of vitality around the body, can empower unwinding, stop pains, fast recovery, and decrease different manifestations of ailment.

Reiki has been around for a huge number of years. The practice was first created in

1922 by a Japanese Buddhist called Mikao Usui, who purportedly showed 2,000 individuals the Reiki strategy during his lifetime. The training spread to the U.S. through Hawaii during the 1940's, and after that to Europe during the 1980's.

Nonetheless, there is no logical proof to help asserts that alleged fundamental energy really exists, nor is there definitive proof that Reiki is valuable for any wellbeing related purpose, as indicated by the NCCIH. Be that as it may, even though Reiki hasn't been certified as a viable medical tool, that doesn't mean it's a hurtful practice.

According to Ann Baldwin, a teacher of physiology at the University of Arizona and a Reiki expert, Reiki can "do no harm," at worst, the practice can do nothing.

As of late, Reiki has been coordinated into numerous social insurance settings, including medical clinics, Baldwin disclosed to Live Science. Also, other scientific studies on the practice proposed that this integral treatment might be important for diminishing tension and torment, relaxing, improving exhaustion and mitigating the side effects of depression, indicating by the Center for Spirituality and Healing at the University of Minnesota (UMN).

Essential Things you MUST Remember Before Reiki

Some Reiki experts and novice tend to forget some things when practicing Reiki. You must be aware of these few basic knowledge that is identified with the act of self-treatment and medications accomplished for other people. With this knowledge, you are better informed about the practice

Reiki Heals What Must Be Healed

The healing is not based on what we want to heal. A few people say that "Reiki is an astute vitality" and that it flows where the recuperating will really occur. The truth is, Reiki is not all about insight, but about its distinctive capacity to restore healing in a place where it was lost. This is overlooked here and there, individuals attempt to force the process, and they feel terrible when Reiki didn't give the results they were seeking after. Actually, this happens to every first-timer – including me.

Reiki will only flow and heal, bringing in harmony the things that must be healed, in a way they can be really get healed – nothing else will occur. Each Reiki expert is only a channel for the vitality and has restricted command over this Reiki power.

Make sure to mend the origin of the problem, and not the manifestations: this is the right expectation and it should be the mindset when you are practicing Reiki. For instance, you may experience an individual with a migraine and do Reiki to bring relief from discomfort. Yet even with the good intention of your heart, the aim must be somewhat unique: to recuperate the source of the pain. At the point when the origin is healed, the manifestations are no more existing.

The side effects may not vanish immediately, so keep that in mind and advise this to the individual who approaches you for Reiki. Try not to be disheartened by this and discontinue doing Reiki, note that occasionally, time is fundamental if the origin of the pain is to regain healing.

The Effects of Reiki is Important to Every Customer

By "customer" I mean any individual who approaches you for Reiki: it can be a relative or a companion who is not giving you a dime for it.

At whatever point you offer Reiki to somebody, make certain to disclose to this individual the idea of Reiki healing process. Clarify that first, Reiki mends not the indications, but the root and center of the issue. The side effects may not vanish immediately, so tell the individual to remain patient. Next, make sure you clarify the idea of "purifying" period after Reiki sessions. Most times, this is really the same as what you have encountered after Reiki attunement, or after concentrated self-practice. There are times when the side effects may become more grounded, which is due to the body connected with its self-healing systems.

Describe what synchronicity is after Reiki sessions. The individual may encounter life changes subsequent to taking at least one Reiki medications and even though these progressions are not out of the ordinary, they might be extremely intense. During the period, synchronicity occurs and that customer may see a lot of signs throughout his life, disclosing to him what changes he should grasp, and what things he ought to dispose of from his/her life. If you fail to explain this prior to the session, the person will be afraid to continue Reiki.

Additionally, ensure that the individual desires are healing. A few people simply would prefer not to heal; there are numerous purposes behind that. Check the customer's aim before you start the treatment. If a person believes that healing is not important to him, the exercise might become useless.

The Reiki Precepts are a Central Part of Reiki

The Five Reiki Precepts are frequently disregarded; this is wrong. But then in all actuality, these statutes are basic aspects of Reiki practice and Reiki can't be truly utilized effectively without incorporating these statutes into the life of the expert. They resemble rules, demonstrating to you the ideal approach to healing, by making changes in five extraordinary fields of life – feelings, considerations, appreciation, self-development and empathy to everything in the world. Reiki medications give you the healing energy, yet the rules show you the way. Also, everybody can utilize these statutes. If you are healing others, it is good to tell them about these precepts.

Usui proposed that the statutes ought to be rehashed (ruminated and thought about upon) every day and every morning, best with your hands in a Gassho mudra.

Rehash these statutes thrice toward the beginning of the day and thrice at night, depending on your needs. You can likewise ponder upon the guidelines and thoroughly consider your life as per these standards.

Most experts believe that the two basic ideas behind Reiki are: self-medications and, precisely, the precepts of Reiki. By coordinating the two components into your day by day life, you are on the way to self-healing.

Music Improves the Practice

Background music during Reiki treatment (or self-treatment) is a good thought. It is a good idea because a piece of nice, delicate music improves the conditions of relaxations and quiets the dawn. You would enjoy the use of music when treating yourself or others. With the music, you send the Reiki vitality effectively, and if you are treating others, they get to experience the effect better. Also, background sounds make you achieve better results from each session.

Yet, recall that the music must be delicate and serene. It is anything but wise to play Heavy Metal. Find out which sounds are most suitable for Reiki sessions. Also, find out which music makes you relaxed normally; this includes the music preference of the person you want to heal.

Additionally, keep in mind that the deeper the relaxation, the deeper your hearing. Therefore, as the exercise progresses, the music might become so loud than when you started; and this can be annoying. Therefore, ensure that the music is calm enough; the ideal approach to do so is to play the music, loosen up for 30 minutes and see what volume works best.

However, you should use legal music to avoid any unfavorable situations. There are sites with free sounds that you can get legally.

Be Cautious About Incenses and Fragrance Oils

Numerous professionals appreciate utilizing incenses or scent oils during Reiki treatment. They give this decent, healing and mystical state of mind. Yet, before picking up just any fragrance, you must keep some things in mind.

To begin with, a few out of every odd individual prefer incenses or oils. Furthermore, regardless of whether the individual like these, it doesn't mean the person in question likes that particular aroma and type you wish to utilize. For instance, there are two kinds of scent oils — characteristic (and costly) and fake (typically toxic). It is advisable to use normal oils.

For incenses, there are two sorts of these too – regular and costly, and fake and poisonous. What's more, there are numerous sorts of these incenses with regards to shape and fixings. Incense sticks with wood powder, stick on a bamboo, cones, pitches or incense powders, all of which performs distinctively.

In all honesty, the ideal approach to buy incenses is to look for them on Etsy, where many individuals handcraft these. Inquire as to whether the incense is 100% organic, which is what you should use. A Buddhist-type incense "Bodhileaf incense" (aff) (stick incenses) are incredible, as well. They are made and delivered in Nepal. Oftentimes, Buddhist associations import and sell them. The natural White Sage or herbs like this can be utilized as incenses, as well.

Try not to use cheap and poisonous incenses that are regularly sold in profound stores. High-quality incenses are great, however once a major organization begins to make incenses, the impact of their work is normally upsetting.

Ensure That Your Client Is Comfortable

You can't disregard your customer's solace. Keep in mind that when an individual rests on a bed, his temperature may appear lower due to the slow progression of the blood. In simpler terms, the person you are healing might get cold since he is not moving. Ensure you have prepared a cover for the individual when this occurs.

Also, the proper position on the bed is important for comfort. If you do Reiki sessions on a regular schedule, it's best to get yourself a back rub table. Put a pad under your head or the person's, for one. Likewise, place a pad or something comparative under the knees, as it will loosen up this locale of the body, as well. Lastly, place a cushion or something comparative under the lower legs – once more, this will enable the body to unwind.

Remember About Self-Treatment

This is significant – regardless of how long you practice Reiki and what number of customers you had previously, despite everything you have to rehearse Reiki yourself. Self-treatment is the most well-known approach to work with Reiki, yet you can likewise learn Japanese systems of contemplation (for instance, from the prescribed The Reiki Sourcebook) and utilize these. There are numerous strategies to look over, for example, Gassho reflection, Joshin Kokyu Ho and so on.

Recuperating and developing yourself is the fundamental component of Reiki practice – which, from multiple points of view, is simply the way improvement and self-mending. Attempt to work with Reiki vitality for at any rate 30 minutes out of every day. Also, remember that sending Reiki to your nourishment or plants is additionally an approach to rehearse.

You're not a Doctor – Don't Play One

In case you're not a specialist of medication, don't diagnose or prescribe anything to people. Try not to propose explicit medicinal issues to your patients. In the event that you see something dangerous that you don't care for (in light of the fact that you've read a couple of restorative books), don't call it, don't discuss it, simply recommend the customer to proceed to visit an expert therapeutic authority.

Frequently, your customer may ask "you touched my liver – do I have liver issues?!" in such or comparable cases, you can just say that you do Reiki dependent on instinct and what you feel where you ought to send Reiki and you don't generally have a clue why you ought to do this with the exception of the way that you feel this is correct. Possibly, you ought to disclose to the customer the strategy of Byosen Reikan Ho.

Try not to Commercialize Practice Too Much

The act of Reiki is intended to heal your own life. However, you should not learn it for the sole purpose of becoming a Reiki expert or educator. Actually, it is not really a good idea to be a Reiki instructor because you might lose your healing while trying to heal others (most especially beginners that do not entirely want to be healed)

Frequently, Reiki will demonstrate to you your actual gifts that have nothing to do with healing. Understand that while it is natural for some people to become Reiki experts, others will continue to struggle with it. Nevertheless, keep in mind that Reiki has a lot to do with healing rather than making money.

Chapter 4: What You Should Know About Reiki As A Beginner

The term "Reiki" simply means the flow of miraculous sign and energy from the atmosphere. It comes from "rei" (universal) and "ki" (life energy) Japanese words. Reiki is a kind of healing energy.

What is Reiki?

Reiki is a Japanese practice with a designation that means "universal life energy." This method is based on the concept that the practitioner can facilitate the flow and smooth transmission of the customer's own spiritual energy through contact or proximity. In the late 1930s, Mrs.

Hawayo Takata brought Reiki largely to the west from Japan. Over time, Takata passed on her knowledge to others, and the technique spread throughout the west.

The physician softly touches the patient with both hands in particular positions during a Reiki session or holds his or her hands slightly above the patient. Typically, Reiki sessions last about an hour. During the session, the practitioner places his or her hands on or over the patient's body in up to 15 distinct traditional hand positions, holding each position for two to five minutes at a moment. The therapy is totally non-invasive and does not require any manipulation of tissue or painful pressure.

How Does it Work?

People who practice Reiki know that there are blocked energy pathways that exemplify pain and disease in the body. The objective of Reiki treatments is to increase energy flow through these blocked or troubled pathways, this reduces pain and increases the natural capacity of the body to battle disease and cure itself. Reiki can assist decrease pain associated with the development of the disease in cancer patients. It can also decrease some of the unpleasant symptoms frequently experienced by patients during cancer therapy such as depression, lack of strength, and vomiting. In addition, Reiki can also enhance the emotional health and perspective of the patient, which may enhance the capacity and readiness of the patient to follow the directions of the physician and stick to therapy protocols.

It is said that Reiki involves transferring universal energy from the palms of the practitioner to their patient. Energy healing has been used in different forms for millennia. Advocates argue that it operates with the body's energy fields. A 2007 study reveals that at least once in the past years, 1 million plus adolescents in the United States (U.S.) attempted Reiki or comparable therapy. It is thought that more than 60 hospitals give patients Reiki services.

Reiki Attunement, What Is It?

The method through which an individual gets the capacity to give Reiki treatments is Reiki attunement. During the Reiki class, the attunement is administered by the Reiki Master. During the attunement, The Reiki Master touches the head, hands, and shoulders and of the person and uses one or more unique relaxation techniques. Attunement energies will flow into the person through the Reiki Master. The Higher Power guides these unique energies and makes changes in the energy pathways of the learners and connects the student to Reiki's source. Since the Higher Power guides the energetic aspect of the tuning, it adjusts for each student to be precisely correct. Some people feel warm in their hands during the tuning, others may see colors or have spiritual beings visions. However, for the tuning to have worked, it is not essential to have an inner experience. Most of it just feels more relaxed.

You're Considering Learning Reiki?

Reiki is a very easy learning method and is not dependent on having any previous experience with healing, meditation or any other type of practice. More than a million individuals from all walks of life have discovered it effectively, the young as well as old. More reason why learning it is so simple is that it's learned without been pre-trained. The capacity to do Reiki is simply transmitted from the teacher through a mechanism called an attunement during a Reiki class to the student. As soon as one receives an attunement, they have the ability to do Reiki and after that whenever one places their hands on themselves or on another person with the intention of doing Reiki, the healing energy will automatically begin flowing.

Starting A Reiki Practice

Whether you're just beginning a Reiki practice to provide Reiki healing for customers or patients in need or you're planning to give Reiki training to teach others how to deliver Reiki treatments, Starting a Reiki company enables you to give a bigger amount of individuals this unique therapy. It may also be a source of income to start a Reiki practice – there is increasing demand for this secure and efficient strategy to Reiki healing.

Just like opening up any other form of company, starting the Reiki practice needs foresight and planning. Once you understand how to begin a Reiki company, healing typically begins dramatically.

Planning to Start Reiki Business

You're going to want to know everything about Reiki first and then find a Reiki Master Teacher to study with. Then you will finish training classes on Reiki, practicing at home and on yourself and potentially family or friends. Before you strike out on your own, it is vital that you get well- rounded schooling in Reiki. It is essential for you to be comfortable with the Reiki energy before providing Reiki services to others.

Where To Practice

Look for a place to treat Reiki. Some districts enable Reiki professionals from their own homes to function. You might prefer to lease a room, maybe share a room with a surgeon, health therapist or massage therapist. Whether you're planning to provide Reiki healing at home or in a leased firm room, the facility needs to provide your customers with privacy and convenience.

Get a Reiki Table

Invest in a nice table for bodywork. If you are unable to afford a fresh one, we're in a digital globe, a search on the internet for quality would do or contact local massage schools for some Reiki tables suggestions that practitioners discovered to be comfortable, portable, and low-cost.

Gain Experience and Build Your Client Base

Develop a client base and acquire expertise by contracting or volunteering in hospitals, nursing homes, hospices, and other facilities where patients may benefit from Reiki medicines. are there any assisting organizations that might profit from your moment with Reiki or volunteering? A position dear to your heart's cause?

Spread the Word

Let others understand you're beginning a practice of Reiki. Ask friends, family and customers or patients with whom you have worked to write testimonials for you to publish or show as printed reviews on your website. Recommendations are always better than advertising that is paid.

Your Reiki Treatments

Treat every client of Reiki as a precious person. It should be slow, meticulous and professional for Reiki treatments. The meeting has everything to do with the client. You are there as a Reiki practitioner to promote a relaxing and well-being atmosphere for your customers. As an additional side advantage to you, Observe up at the end of the session with each client to ensure that the healing or relaxation method continues after the end of the Reiki session and to offer any help to questions they may have. The longer you exercise Reiki and experience its advantages, the more you will certainly be motivated to continue your Reiki education. To learn more about Reiki techniques or brush up on your current Reiki abilities, attend Reiki training classes. It's simple to start a Reiki exercise once all the details are known. Finding a regular exercise that takes you away from ' day to day ' is so essential to remind you that it's all right. ' said by Ian Tucker in Your Simple Path – Find happiness in every step.

The quote describes what Reiki is – the touch of healing. To enhance one's health and quality of life is a life force energy. In its recovery, it has a spiritual element. For ' Higher Power, ' ' Rei ' is the Japanese term and ' ki ' is the energy of life force. That is to say, Reiki is an ' energy of life force spiritually guided. '

Time Taken while learning Reiki

On a weekend, a starting Reiki class is taught. The class may last for one or two days. I consider at least six to seven hours for the minimum moment needed. Together with the attunement, it's essential to show the student how to treat and how to exercise treatment in the environment.

Putting Reiki in perspective

Reiki is an interaction of a person individually. It is unlikely that anyone who does not believe the therapy will experience any benefit of it. One of Reiki's main principles is that it would not cause damage because it is applied without tampering or force but only using a light touch, for individuals with pain, restricted mobility, or extreme weakness, it is recommended.

About Reiki Hand Positions – the Basics

Going in for your first therapy, these are the positions that you can usually expect to use because they are typical of most therapy sessions. Every other position is designed to balance the energies in that region and remove stuck energies so you can start relaxing, Reduce stress and allow your body to rest and heal and work better. If you need special attention to be given to one region, let your physician know. Your physician will often be able to detect regions within the hand positions that need additional attention that may not even have been revealed to you.

Positions of Hand During Reiki Application

In Reiki, there are basic typical and basic hand positions taught in Reiki certification classes that are used to encourage energy distribution and healing to different fields of the body. During a Reiki therapy, more time may be spent on one region than another depending on your specific health problem. This article, commonly speaking, highlights the fundamental Reiki hand positions. Some of the hand positions may be omitted and/or during a session may happen in a distinct order. Depending on your individual requirements, variations can also be made on these roles.

Expectation During Treatment With Reiki

A customer rests comfortably on a massage table during a Reiki session or is sometimes sitting on a chair. There is no tissue manipulation occurring in massage or bodywork, but only a very gentle pressure of the hand. Unlike massage treatment, during a Reiki session, you are always completely clothed. The session generally takes place in silence with a relatively no conversation, unless you want to tell your practitioner something, then it's essential that you do it quickly. Your Reiki practitioner can play relaxing background music or sounds of nature. If you're awkward or comfortable, or the music is distracting, for instance, or you prefer to skip some Reiki hand position, just let your physician know before or during your session.

The Reiki "Touch"

Reiki is conducted either with very gentle, static pressure from the practitioner's hands on traditional hand-positioned fields, or with a few inches above your body with their hands. In either case, Reiki works almost as well, so if you prefer not to be touched directly with any or all of the hand positions and prefer the hovering method, please let your practitioner know before or during your session, preferably before the session. During a Reiki session, sensitive or private regions will never be affected. Even if in a delicate or private region you have a health problem, it is against the Code of Ethics of a Reiki Professional Practitioner to physically touch personal or sensual regions. Your Reiki practitioner wants you to feel refreshed and be comfortable as possible while enjoying this timeless Japanese energy technique work for stress reduction, relaxation, and well-being.

Here are some of the most popular general hand positions in the Reiki session that you could encounter:

Position A

Palms are put on your forehead lightly and/or the fingers of the practitioner may cup your eyes softly.

Position B

The physician could also put his hands on the edges of your temples and face soothingly.

Position C

The practitioner's hands may cradle your head as his or her hands rest on the table.

Position D

Reiki can be provided softly to your jawline or throat region.

Position E

The right or left hand of the practitioner might well swing or be positioned near your throat or above your collarbone, while your other hand may swing or be positioned above your chakra core which is around your heart region.

Position F

Hands can be softly put on your pelvic area.

Position G

The physician can put his hands on your solar plexus or mid-abdomen

Position H

The practitioner can put his hands on your lower middle abdomen a few inches below your navel.

Position I

A physician may preferably give Reiki to your knees and/or wrists or feet. If the physician feels they can benefit you, these are alternative positions. Or they can just move on to your back's side positions.

Position J

The physician may ask you to turn on your belly with your head in a face cradle or softly resting on one side if you are on a massage table. The hands of the practitioner are softly put and rested on your shoulder blade region.

Position K

Hands are shifted below your shoulder blades or the middle back area of the body.

Position L

The physician moves his hands to apply gentle pressure on your lower back with soft hand placement.

Once all the fundamental positions and/or variants are covered and energies are lifted or balanced, the physician can move his hands over your body in a sweeping movement to clean your energy field from any remaining energy residue, Leaving you clean, feeling happy and strengthening your well-being path.

Afterward

Feel free to keep your body hydrated after your session for 24 hours and take some time after your session, even just a few minutes, to observe peace and quietness. Try to enable yourself to gain gratitude from your greater self for caring so eloquently for your body, mind, and spirit sometime after your workout or perhaps later in the evening before bed and to appreciate your enhanced state of well-being and peace.

Can I Treat Myself?

Yes, you could also treat yourself as well as others once you have got the attunement. This is one of Reiki's distinctive characteristics. I've heard Reiki can be performed from a distance to others.

How Is This Going To Work?

You are provided 3 Reiki symbols in Reiki II (Deeper Level). The attunement to Reiki II empowers these symbols. One of these symbols is for remote healing by using an image of the individual you want to send Reiki to or by writing the name of the individual on a piece of paper or simply thinking about the individual and activating the remote symbol, No matter where they are, you can send Reiki to them. They might be thousands of miles away, but that doesn't matter. The energy from Reiki is going to go to them and treat them. You can also send Reiki to disasters or global leaders, and they will also be aided by Reiki energy.

How many Reiki training levels are there?

There are four levels in Reiki's Usui / Tibetan scheme taught by the Center. These include the first, the second, the Advanced and the Master.

Can A Reiki Individual Be Earning A Living From It?

If you put your heart into it, coupled with teaching courses, you can create a Reiki practice that can generate a periodic revenue. This is a very satisfying way of earning a living.

Can One Be Licensed For Reiki Activity And Teaching?

At this moment, there is no government licensing programs. However, for Reiki

educators, However, there are International Centers and Teachers Guidebook available from these Center, the Centers have a licensing program.

Does Reiki treatment cover insurance?

Insurance companies are just beginning to recognize Reiki. Although not many of them cover Reiki treatments, there are some.

Can nurses Nurses or yoga teachers take Reiki courses?

Courses conducted by Reiki teachers' centers are endorsed to be offered to nurses, massage therapists and athletic trainers with adequate training and certificates.

Reiki lineage

Reiki is a method that is continuously transferred from professor to student. If you have Reiki, then you will be part of a sequence of educators that will lead back to the Reiki system founder that you are practicing. The lineage would lead back to Dr. Usui in the case of the Usui Reiki lineage.

Chapter 5: Reiki Symbols And Their Unique Uses

Many Reiki Masters consider the Reiki symbols holy and persist in the old Reiki tradition that they must be kept secret. The symbols should only be available to those who have been initiated at the Reiki 2 level. Many people today feel that this approach is no longer relevant as the symbols have been described in many books and freely available on the Internet. However, it is also believed the Reiki symbols and the information that can be read about them are of little value on their own.

In different tests it has been proven that the symbols have little or no use before a Reiki initiation. Students with no Reiki experience (but with psychic abilities) have been asked to memorize the symbols and then use them. The results differ from a control group will had the Reiki 2 initiation. The conclusion has been that it is the Reiki initiation as suchthat gives the Reiki symbols their power.The Reiki symbols are like keys which open doors to a higher mind. You can also see them as buttons, when you press the button, you automatically get a result. The symbols trigger a belief or intention built into the symbols to help the user to get the results intended. The different symbols also quickly connect the user to the universal life force. When a Reiki Master does an attunement and shows the symbols to the student, the form of the symbol is impressed in the mind and merges with the metaphysical energies it represents. When a Reiki practitioner draws, thinks about or visualizes a symbol, it instantly connects to the energies it represents.

Today, there are many different forms of Reiki, and some have incorporated their own symbols in the initiations. In "traditional" Reiki, there are three Reiki symbols given during the Reiki attunement. They are: The Power Symbol (Choku Rei) The Mental/Emotional Symbol (Sei He Ki) The Distance Symbol (Hon Sha Ze Sho Nen). The Reiki symbols are partly based on the Japanese writing system, Kanji. The symbols should be drawn or visualized as they have been taught during a Reiki 2 attunement. As more and more people get attuned to Reiki, this means that there can be a great number of variations between symbols taught by different Masters. This is not really a problem as there is not 100% right or wrong way to draw them. The Reiki symbols given to a student will work however they look, as they incorporate the intention and the connection to the metaphysical energies they represent. Having said that, it is our belief that it is essential to keep as much as is physically possible to the original symbols as distortions over time are symptomatic of our need for healing in the first place.

THE REIKI POWER SYMBOL OF CHOKU REI

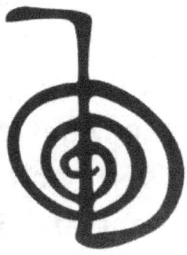

The general meaning of Choku Rei (pronounced Cho-Koo-Ray) is "place the power of the universe here". The Power Symbol can be used to increase the power of Reiki, or it can be used for protection. See it as a light switch that has the intention to instantly boost your ability to channel Reiki. Draw or visualize the symbol in front of you and you will have instant access to more healing energies. Choku Rei also gives the other symbols more power when they are used together. The symbol can be used at any time during a treatment, but it is especially effective if it is used at the beginning of a session or when used at the end of a session to close and seal off the Reiki energies. Remember it is always your intention that governs what happens. If you want to add new functions to the Power Symbol, then just have a clear statement and intention of what you want the symbol to do and it will do it for you.

Uses of Choku rei

Increase the power of your healing abilities; use it as a light switch. (Draw or visualize Choku Rei in front of you or draw it in your hands if you want). * You can focus the Reiki energies (like a looking glass) on a specific point of the body. (Draw the symbol directly on the spot being treated).

Increase the power of the other symbols. (Draw it before drawing the other symbols). * One can use the Power Symbol to close the space around the recipient.

(Draw it above the body with the intention of sealing the process).

The Power Symbol can be used to spiritually clean a room from negative energies. (Draw or visualize the Symbol on all the walls, ceiling and floor with the intention to protect and energize the room).

You can clean crystals and other objects from negative energies. (Draw the Power Symbol above or on the Crystal/object with the intention of cleansing it and restoring it to its original state. Hold the object in your hands and give it Reiki (or send it Reiki from a distance if the object is far away or too big to hold).

Protect yourself from negative energies (from people you treat or from people you meet). Draw or visualize the Reiki Power Symbol in front of you with the intention of being totally protected.

Protect yourself, your children, your spouse, your house and other things you value. (Draw Choku Rei directly on the objects/person you want to protect with the intention to protect him/her from harm. Since Reiki works on all different levels of existence, it will naturally also given protection on all levels of existence.

There are no limits to what you can do. The power is all in your mind - let your clear intention guide the function of the symbols.

THE REIKI Mental/Emotional Symbols- Sei He Ki

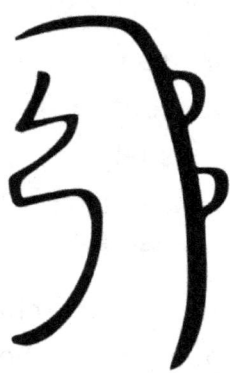

Sei He Ki (pronounced Say-Hay-Key) has a general meaning of "God and Man become one". The Mental/Emotional symbol brings together the "brain and the body". It helps people to bring to the surface and release the mental/emotional causes of their problems. Many people (even doctors) are starting to realize that many of our ailments are based on mental and emotional imbalances.

The symbol works to focus and harmonize the subconscious with the physical side. It can be used to help with emotional and mental healing. It balances the left and right side of the brain and gives peace and harmony. It is also very effective at relationship problems. The symbol can also be used on diverse problems like nervousness, fear, depression, anger, sadness etc.

Uses of See He Ki

The symbols can be used to help overcome misuse of drugs, alcohol, smoking, etc.

Sei He Ki can be used to lose weight.

The symbol can be used to find things that you have misplaced. (Draw the symbol in front of you and ask for help in finding the object. Let go of trying, the answer will soon pop up).

Sei He Ki can be used to improve your memory when reading or studying. (Draw the symbol on each page as you read it with the intention of remembering the important parts).

Add the symbol with doing healing (normal or distance) as this can help the healing process. Many physical problems have mental/emotional roots.

The Mental/Emotional Symbol, Sei He Ki, has to do with Yin and Yang and the balance between the two sides of the brain. The left part of the symbol represents Yang and our left side of the brain (logic, structure and linear thinking etc).

The right side of this symbol represents Yin and our right side of the brain (fantasy, feelings, intuition, etc).

Chapter 6: Time For Change

I remember going to walk in my local park the day after my attunement. The colours were more vibrant and all I could hear were the sounds of nature. I had never taken notice of these things before. I became more aware of everything around me and the beauty of nature. I recognised the sounds of the different birds, including to my surprise, a Woodpecker. This has continued up till now, all these years later. Until then a park had just been a place to walk my dog. I would also walk quickly to get from A to B, so this was something new for me. While I was walking through the park, I felt my hands buzzing as the energy switched on. I looked around me to see who needed reiki but could see no one else.

When I got home, I was walking round the house giving reiki to all my plants. It was if a light had been turned on. I felt I had to give energy to everything. I especially decided to test it by using on one of my tall plants that was due to be binned thinking it was too far gone to be saved. Imagine my delight when after three days it started to look better. After three weeks you would not have known it had ever been a sick plant. In fact, it became so healthy that in the end it towered above its companion plant. How I loved my reiki. The use of reiki is limitless. It can be used for so much.

When I mentioned the time out walking in the park to my teacher, he advised that as there was only me who had been in the park, then the reiki must have been meant for me. I have since found if this happens, all I do is put my hands in my pockets and then I can feel this wonderful energy flowing through me. It's something that I always pass on to my students too now.

I was to get a big surprise though as I found I was able to help others, but not my own back problem, after being trained in level one. I found this frustrating. The interesting thing was my friend, who I had never felt anything from when receiving Reiki, was now able to give such strong Reiki that she was able to help my back whenever I needed it. I remember one time when I had a funeral to go to and my back went big time and I could not stand up. After sitting with her hands on my back for 30 minutes I was able to get through not only the funeral but the wake afterwards. I was very confused about now feeling it from my friend but not being able to do this for myself. I had gone through Usui level one expecting to have the power to help myself and it had not happened. This was to be explained to me later.

Part of the level one training is being told of the Reiki principles that we should try to live by, and I have incorporated these into my life. It is amazing that just changing your mind set can make such a difference in your life. I think that even if those not practising reiki abided by these ideals that the world would be a much happier place.

The Five Principles of Reiki

Just for today, do not worry. Worry changes nothing. If it has already happened, you cannot change it. If it is in the future it may not happen.

Just for today, do not anger. Anger only hurts you. Take a step back or walk away from the situation / conversation.

Just for today, be kind to all people. Having respect for others allows you to have greater respect for yourself. I always tell students that even if someone has upset them, they should send love in that direction.

Earn your living honestly. Living your life this way means you are living as you should. I know if I did something wrong it would come back to bite me!

Show gratitude to every living thing. Once you try,

you can always find reasons to be Grateful. Everything living thing has a purpose on Earth, so we should be grateful for them being hShow gratitude to every living thing.

I am seen by many people now as a calm person who is not quick to anger. This was a big learning curve for me especially as my life was not so good up to that point. I will give you a laugh though. I am so conscious of the honesty part that one Christmas at work we were doing a Secret Santa and had written up three things we might like bought for us. One thing I love is Yankee candles, so this was on my list. I then heard someone in the office was selling these cheaper than normal and asked why. Apparently, they had fallen off the back of a lorry. I then worried that someone would get me one and I would not be able to use it just in case it was one of those. Luckily, I got a totally different make of candle, so I could relax and enjoy it when Santa came.

One of the interesting things I have found with reiki is you do not know where it will take you when you start out. Many people stop after level one as this is all they need. It improves people's lives in so many ways that they are happy with the first level and do not feel the need to take it forward. I love that after one day's training it can make such a difference for people. Learning reiki has taught me more than anything, to live in the present. Of course, that does not stop us making long term goals, but it does make you appreciate where you are now.

I can only say that over time thoughts kept coming into my mind again and again about level two. I had not expected that I would want to go on to the next level, but it seems that I was being directed to do this as there came a time I could not stop thinking of level two. I decided to save up for this and see what I was meant to be taught. I strongly believe that if anything keeps coming back into your mind it is for a reason. Throughout my years with reiki this has happened time and again so now I always act on the thoughts.

Level Two

A few months later I went to the same teacher, David Tyrrell, to be trained to level two. Again, this was only a very small class and I mentioned to him that I felt confused that reiki level one had not helped me but enabled me to help others. People were saying the energy felt very strong when receiving from me, but it was not helping my back at all. He then asked me if anyone had mentioned that the way

I behaved or talked had changed? He told me that he had noticed a big change in me. After thinking about this I said that yes there was a difference. Before level one everything was going wrong in my life and I was anxious for much of the time. I realised how much happier I was with my life now. I was astonished when he told me the energy would go to where it was needed most, not where I had expected or wanted it to go to. It had been working all this time on my mind and I found that I was now a much more positive person than I had been before. I had learned my first lesson. This has been proved time and time again to me since that period when I have treated both myself and clients. Often the energy goes where the client did not expect but when we meet up again, I am advised it was the right thing for them at that time. It may be that someone has stomach aches. Sometimes the energy will concentrate on the head. In those cases, the stomach problem was caused by stress from what was going on in the persons mind.

I was also of the mind-set that if two things had gone wrong, I was just waiting for the third bad thing to happen. How many of us think this way? I hear this, especially in the workplace. If the day started off bad, I would hear people say the rest of the day would continue in the same way. This had now changed for me. I realised it was all about mindset and that after a bad start to the day, it could only get better! This is a much better way of looking at any situation. I always said that if you had a bad call it was a one off. There is no reason to believe that every call after that would be the same. Why do people think that way?

So, in the end reiki level one had turned out to be a positive experience for me. It may seem strange, but it has completely changed the way I see life. Nothing is insurmountable in my life now. I know that I am in the right place at the right time and there is no reason to get stressed. Level one had concentrated on my mind rather than my back and for that I am very grateful.

One thing that had been wrong in my life during that time had been my roof which had been leaking for a while. I had paid three companies to try to fix it with no success. This had me very worried as water was coming into the house and damaging the walls inside. I had not realised, but after training in level one my whole mind-set had changed. Now instead of being anxious I had the attitude of "It's okay, everything will turn out fine" and I did not worry. The roof did eventually get fixed and out of that I got a new Therapy space in my attic to chill out which a friend built for me.

Another thing happened around this time. I had written a blog and I advised that I no longer watched the news on TV but did view it as writing on my laptop. This way you can read without the emotional embellishment that the reporters add to their scripts. After I mentioned this way of thinking to a friend, he thought the same and said if you were meant to hear any news it would come to you at the right time. The very next day I logged into my BT Yahoo site and it had all changed. The sites that I had on there to give me news had disappeared! Instead of the BBC news and my local Newspaper pages it was now blank. After a few minutes of trying to get them back on again I sat back for a moment and had a light bulb moment. A higher source had decided I did not need to see any news at all at this moment in time.

Since then the only time I catch any news is if I switch on the radio and it comes on. I immediately change channel, so I do not have my positive mental attitude decreased. I find even listening to a few seconds saddens me as it's usually bad news. I did have a couple of days of wanting my fix, but this has now gone, and

I am amazed how much lighter I feel now. I have now not watched television or listened to the news for 7 years!

The most amazing thing that I have found recently is many more people are thinking the same way in wanting to stay positive and not be pulled down by negative news. I spoke to someone recently who said he has not seen or heard the news in years too. It's as if a shift is taking place. In actual fact I have been finding a lot more sites that I am being drawn to that are full of good news stories instead. In these days of social media, you get lots of news stories popping up. As I don't trust a lot of what I see, if I'm interested, I do my own research. One of the things you should always do is check the source before sharing news items. Even then you may find the source to be corrupted. Many of the news stories are there to instil fear into us all. It's also important to be aware that what you are seeing may be manipulated. We have all seen the same people that pop up at different war zones!

It's important to be aware that more often good things happen than bad. It seems though, that bad stories make people read newspapers and watch the news on T.V. Since I made the decision to stop watching television it was the best thing for me at that time and it still is.

Chapter 7: Heal Yourself

And so we begin using the art of Reiki to heal yourself. Because the universe's life force is flowing through everyone and everything at all times, using Reiki on yourself does not require any special effort or particular choreography. The art of Reiki treatments are simple to place your hands-on certain parts of your body in order to allow the energy to move and flow between the two touching places. Remember, the energy is already there. The energy is already flowing. You are simply attempting to direct it. You are simply attempting to channel it. You are not the energy. You are simply a conduit and our attempting to make it flow more freely in particular areas.

The way you go about channeling energy is by putting your hands in specific positions on your own body. You do not need any special knowledge about anatomy. Nor do you need to know exactly what part of your own body is most in need. The universal energy is omnipotent and all-knowing. The life force will move to where it is most needed on its own. There is no right or wrong way to place your hands upon yourself. These are simply suggestions and can be modified or experimented with at any time, especially upon yourself.

There are 10 different general hand placements that we will discuss using on yourself:

Face

Head

Neck

Chest

Stomach

Shoulders

Back

Hips

Legs

Feet

Face

Much like if you were washing your face with your hands place your palms over your face, your fingers over your eyes, your eyes closed and breathe. Move your hands up, caressing your fingertips over your forehead to the top of your hairline and bringing your hands down along the side of your face, letting your fingertips move down around your temples, feeling over your cheekbones, down to where your jawline starts and across to the middle of your chin. Bring your fingertips to your nose, letting the flat pads of your fingers lay against your cheeks and bring your hands around in a small circle letting your fingertips end up on your lips. Feel free to continue moving your hand around your face, or simply letting your hands lay still on your face. Because our faces and the skin in this area is so sensitive, please take care to do everything very gently. Make sure your eyes are closed. Be sure to not poke yourself in the eye. Go as slowly as you need.

Let your fingers come back to your jaw bone where it meets your neck and lay one hand along each side of your jaw. Feel the curve of your jaw bone in the palm of your hand. Then slowly but firmly press your fingertips into your jaw bone and gently drag your fingers down to your chin. Turning your fingers to face towards your ears and bringing your wrists together to touch at your chin, simply rest your hands on your jaw. Now cross your arms and place your right hand over your left jaw bone and your left hand over your right jaw bone, repeating the previous movement of your fingers down to your chin.

Head

Cupping your hands over your ears and moving your hands towards your face half an inch, let your fingers rest around your temples. Bring your hands toward the top of your head, letting your pinkies lineup along your hairline. Gently let your hands fall down and around the back of your head as if you were rinsing water out of your hair. Clasp your fingers around each other at the base of your skull, letting your headrest in your hands for a moment. Then unlock your fingers and bring your hands back up to just behind your ears. Again, feel free to go as slowly as necessary. You may or may not want to use more pressure on your scalp. Feel free to use your fingertips to get beneath the hair and to the skin on your head, although this is not necessary. Take care while placing your hands on your head not to move your neck too much. You do not need to move your neck to reach any places in particular. You also do not want to strain your neck doing this.

Neck

Very gently place one hand over the front of your neck, making sure not to apply any pressure or squeeze whatsoever. Feel your pulse underneath your finger. Gently put your other hand on the back of your neck, allowing your fingers to touch around your neck if possible. If not possible, do not force this. It is not necessary. Release your hands and turning your fingers toward your ears place both of your hands on either side of your neck, with your wrists touching in front of you, just underneath your chin. Release and cross your arms in front of you, allowing your right hand to wrap around the left side of your neck and your left hand to wrap around to the right side of your neck.

Now allow your hands to continue traveling down your neck and across your collarbone. Feel your décolletage extend out to your shoulders. Then bring your hands back across to the opposite side allowing your left hand to end up on your left shoulder and your right hand to end up on your right shoulder, if that is possible for you. If you cannot reach or are not flexible enough to touch your shoulders, that is quite all right.

Chest

Laying each hand on the top of your chest just below the collarbone, keep your hand flat, but do not apply pressure or push down on your chest. As much as you are comfortable feel free to move your hands across your chest. Make sure to place at least one hand right between your breasts, as this is where the heart chakra resides. Move your hands down further and place each palm over either side of your rib cage. Allow your hands to fall down the sides of you as far as is comfortable for your flexibility. Then cross your arms and place your right hand over your left rib cage and your right hand over your left rib cage starting from your far side moving your hands in toward each other meeting at the center of your chest. With your fingertips, drag your fingers up your center chest towards your neck and back down, using just your fingertips.

Because your chest takes up a wide swath of your body, feel free to spend as much or as little time here as you would like. Using your hands to go up and down the center of your chest repeatedly is a good practice that you will find has a lot of soothing qualities.

Stomach

Laying your hands on your stomach, this is another area that will do well with up and down emotions over the center of your stomach. The stomach will also benefit from using circular motions, specifically clockwise motions over your digestive system. It is especially helpful to make tracks across your stomach from side-to-side two or three times. You can do this in many ways. You can put both hands next to each other, side-by-side, starting on your left side and dragging both of your hands across your stomach over the middle and down to your right side, and then going back from right to left. You can do these two or three times. Or you could start with one hand on each side, and simultaneously move them toward each other and then across to the opposite side. Again, going back and forth two or three times.

However, some people find this to be uncomfortable, especially after having eaten. In that case, feel free to simply lay your hands statically on your stomach, without movement. Another great exercise to do here is by letting your middle fingers touch each other tip-to-tip, and laying those right over your navel. Let your hands lay here, right over the center of your stomach for a few moments. No movement is necessary.

Shoulders

If you are lying down, you may want to sit up or stand in order to do your shoulders.

Reaching up and over your own shoulders as much as is comfortable for your level of flexibility, place your hands on your shoulders and run them as far down your back as possible. With your hands on your back, run your hands back and forth from side to side, applying as much pressure with your fingertips as you would like. Release your hands, cross your arms in front of you, and place each hand on the opposite shoulder feel free to reach as far behind you as possible, although this may be very difficult. Move your hands over your shoulders and down your arms ending up with your hands holding each other. You can also take one arm at a time to reach the back of your shoulder blades. Lifting your right arm straight above you, bend at the elbow so that your hand is now behind your head. Put your left hand on your right elbow and allow it to push your right hand farther down your back. Again, this is important to note that you should not do anything that hurts or is uncomfortable. You do not need to reach farther down your shoulder blades then is comfortable for you.

Back

To reach your back, you can simply place your hands behind your back, and use either the back of your hands if that is all that is feasible for you based on your flexibility, or if you are able to turn your palms towards your back, even for just a small portion of area, you can do that as well. In your back, a great motion would be going up and down your spine, making sure not to apply any pressure, and repeating this motion a few times. The same as with your stomach, you can also move your hands back and forth from side to side across your back as much as is possible for you. An important area to try to reach on your back would be your low back area. Placing your right hand on your right low back and your left hand on your left low back, allowing your fingertips to point towards your buttocks, let your hands rest here for a moment over your root chakra.

Hips

From there you can simply move your hands further down to rest on your hip bones. As always, do whatever is most comfortable for you, because this is simply for yourself. Move your hands further back as far as you can feel your hip bones around you, and is comfortable for your amount of flexibility. Moving your hands back and forth over your hip bones two or three times. Move your hands lower about one inch in order to feel the very top of the leg where it connects to your hip. Again move your hands back and down as far as comfortable for you. Then turn your wrists as much as possible pointing your fingertips down toward your toes and move your hands from side to side. Much like with your stomach, you can do this a couple of ways. Placing your hand side by side and moving from left to right together, or starting with one hand on either side and crossing opposite of each other.

Legs

While performing Reiki on yourself, this is the point at which if you were laying, you will most likely need to sit up. You could also always perform it on yourself while sitting in a chair. In order for you to reach your own legs, get into whatever position is most comfortable for you. Placing your hands on the top of your thighs, feel free to move your hands up, down, and all-around your upper legs. Make sure to take turns using the opposite hand on the opposite leg. It is best to take some time using both hands on your left leg, as well as using both hands on your right leg. As much as possible based on how you are sitting, standing, or laying, reach as much as possible to feel the underside of your thighs, as well.

Next, you will move to your own knees. Feel free to cup one hand over each knee and move it around in a circular motion. Again, make sure to use your right hand on your left knee and your left hand on your right knee as well. This helps to move energy across your body. While you are at your knee, cup both hands around each knee for a moment. Then use your left hand on your right knee and your right hand on your right hip in order to channel energy from these two areas of major movement. After a moment, be sure to switch, with your right hand on your left knee and your left hand on your left hip.

Moving your hands down your calf, again going as slowly as you need and crossing your hands over to the opposite side as well as using both hands on each side. Do the same as you just did for your knee and hip you should do with your knee and ankle. Putting your left hand on your right ankle and your right hand on your right knee, pause here for a moment. Release and switch to do the same on the other side.

Feet

For your feet, because they contain so many bones and so much energy, even though they may seem small, you will want to take the time to truly cover all of your feet. Placing your palms on the top of your foot and moving it down towards your toes, and then back up again towards your ankle a few times. You will also want to lay your palms flat on the top of your feet moving your hands from side to side across the width of your foot from your pinky toe to your big toe and down over the arch of your foot and bringing your fingertips around your ankle back to your heel. You can use slight pressure with your fingertips if it is comfortable, if not there is no need. Starting with your fingertips on your toes drag your hands back across the sides of your feet and back around your ankle, cupping your heel. Lifting your foot up, place your flat palm against the bottom of your foot, moving your hand up and down. Wrap your palm around your toes moving your hand back and forth across all of your toes. Cup the bottom of your heel into your hand rotating your hand around in a circular motion. Using both of your hand's cup either side of your ankle and rotate your hands as much as possible around your ankle.

Chapter 8: Benefits Of Reiki

Before you begin to practice Reiki healing, you might be wondering, "What benefit can I get from it?"

You have already learned what Reiki means, how the world has received it, where it came from, as well as what its other forms are. So, what's in it for you? Will it help you in some way? Are they the real deal?

You bet they are! When Dr. Mikao Usui created this healing system, he had the determination to create one that could be beneficial for everyone.

The Well-Known Benefits of Reiki

Reiki has been known to provide many benefits to the people who seek to learn and master it. For years, they have been praised by those who have received them as well. Here are some well-known advantages of Reiki.

1. It gives you a radiance that flows through you

When you are practicing Reiki, you can't help but feel radiance flow through you. You will feel this wonderful glow that enlightens you. It makes you feel like you are on top of the world, and you want it to last. To put it simply, Reiki helps you boosts your mood. This means that you will go from being a little down to feeling happier. After all, you are cultivating the energy from within, so you will no doubt feel your body differently.

2. It helps you get through the negativities in life

By doing Reiki healing, you will be able to navigate through the negativity in your life. Whether you feel stressed or stumped, Reiki will get you through these issues. It can even be used as a way to treat depression. Aside from this, you will also manage to face the negative emotions that have been plaguing you with an energy you may have never thought you have.

3. It helps you achieve better focus

One of Reiki's benefits is allowing you to achieve better focus. It helps you cleanse your mind, so you will slowly learn to be more comfortable with yourself. When this happens, you will have a considerable amount of focus and get the things you have meant to finish faster without fail.

Reiki also helps you banish the negativities and distractions that cloud your mind. So, you can get the solution that you have been trying to look for to get through a task by practicing Reiki.

4. It aids in your spiritual growth

Whether you are religious or not, Reiki can help with your spiritual growth. It does not even have to be referred to as such; it is more about growing and evolving as a person. As you have learned earlier, Reiki is spiritual in nature, so you will feel a more significant presence reside within you. You may even be able to appreciate the celestial side of life. Though it may not make some people suddenly turn to God or other deities for help right away, Reiki can still be a good step towards appreciating the spirituality we all have in ourselves.

5. you will be able to relax

It can be challenging to relax these days. With all the responsibilities and hardships that you may go through in life, it is a challenge to find a way to chill.

When you do Reiki, however, you will be able to relax because you will feel a peace of mind that you normally do not get if you let other things bother you. you will also manage to stop minding the chaos around you. While it won't happen in a snap, give it more time, and relaxation will be a breeze.

6. It improves health symptoms and conditions

While Reiki is seen as pseudoscience by many experts, many individuals who have given it a try have found that it can treat some of their symptoms, such as tension, insomnia, and headache. The reason is that the relaxation and calmness that both come from the Reiki healing methods can improve a person's overall health. While some may point out that there is not any hard evidence related to it, the testimonials from patients and practitioners say otherwise.

7. It helps you see yourself in a whole new way

Another benefit of Reiki is that you are able to see yourself on a whole new light. How you have perceived yourself before doing Reiki will change when you begin your journey. You will learn some aspects of yourself that you have never thought you have. It will also get you through the questions that still linger in your mind. This can be seen as a boost to the fourth benefit above because you will also be able to wake up your spiritual side this way.

8. It can help you be one with nature

As Reiki involves energy, you will have no issues with being one with nature. After all, the practice helps you understand various forms of energy all around you, so feeling nature's energy will be beneficial for you. For that reason, you can take a walk in the park because you will be happy to see nature in a whole new light.

9. It can give you better sleep

This is one well-known benefit that many individuals always point out because sleep is always an issue for them before learning about Reiki. By practicing this healing method, though, all the toxins can be detoxified from your body. You will be able to relax and become one with yourself. You can finally sleep in peace and not have to worry about insomnia anymore.

10. It can help you complement other medical therapies and treatments

Another great benefit of Reiki healing is that it can complement the other holistic treatments that you may already be doing, such as yoga and Pilates. You can think of the practice as a way to feel your energy within yourself so that you can use it to boost your performance. So, whether you are doing yoga to be more flexible or doing cardio exercises to lose weight, Reiki can be a nice little method to practice to keep yourself up and running with a glow.

11. It can help you alleviate pain physically and mentally

Reiki can also be beneficial when you are dealing with physical or mental pain. Now, it doesn't mean that you will instantly be able to heal at once, but it can undoubtedly give you a headstart. Also, with the Reiki methods you will learn down the line, you can slowly encourage yourself to let your body improve itself. In time, you will feel the healing within.

12. It can help you manage your emotions

With Reiki healing, you can manage your emotions. For all of us, emotions are part of our lives. From happiness to anger, they all have different effects on us. It can be a bit daunting to manage your feelings when they manifest from within; that's why you need to learn how to control them when you master Reiki. This doesn't mean that you can flip the switch and expect your emotions to go away in an instant, but you can learn to accept them and be able to decide what can be done when you feel a certain emotion.

13. It can help you find balance

Another benefit that you can gain from Reiki healing is that it will help you find inner balance. When it comes to our energy, we may find imbalances occur within ourselves. They can be a bit disruptive and won't be beneficial. When you practice Reiki, though, you will be able to rebalance your energy and find the direction you have been looking for.

14. It can help you be comfortable with yourself

Reiki will help you feel comfortable with yourself. The reason is that you will learn to cultivate the energy that only you can have, as well as dig deep and find out who you are.

15. It will help you learn how to channel energy

Reiki is also beneficial when it comes to learning how to channel energies. Even when you are not moving, you are cultivating energy as you breathe in and out.

Before learning about Reiki, you may not have much to do with the energy. But when you get comfortable with Reiki healing, you will know what to do with it and be able to use it in a variety of ways.

16. You can learn to heal yourself and others

Finally, Reiki can teach you how to treat yourself. As you learn to be comfortable in letting a practitioner help you out in the first few sessions, you can try the techniques that are built for one person. You can even choose to become a practitioner and apply what you have learned to become better at it and heal others.

Healing Effects Through Qi

While Reiki may not be familiar to many, the energy property can be referred to as "qi." In Chinese culture, qi is known as a vital part of any living thing. From humans to animals, there is qi. To cultivate it, there's a method that many citizens in China and the rest of the world have been keeping alive for many years.

Officially classified as qi gong, this alternative healing method allows you to do a series of coordinated body movements, meditation exercises, and breathing techniques that help you balance the qi within you. It originates from China and is different from Reiki because of how the methods are administered, as well as the movements involved. If you must know, Reiki has lesser moves than qi gong.

The common denominator of the two practices is the fact that they promote energy healing. With that idea, what are the healing effects that a person can feel when getting a qi going session?

1. Reduce Stress Level

Just like Reiki, qi gong can help you reduce your stress levels. As you begin to become one with yourself, you will feel all the things that have been stressing you out start to fade away, giving you a new kind of light and radiance. What you are feeling is your qi rising from underneath the negativity.

2. Reduce Pain

Much like Reiki, qi gong helps you get lesser pain since you will be doing movements that have you be comfortable with your body. You will start to feel the physical and mental illness that's been cultivating will all be banished away when you have finally developed the qi within your body.

3. Boost Heart Health

Qi gong also aims to promote better heart health. Because of the yoga-like movements included, you will feel that your qi begins to strengthen all parts of your body, including your heart. When you are finally done, you will feel your heart become stronger.

4. Achieve Energy Balance

Through qi, you will be able to sense your energy going back to equilibrium. It is similar to Reiki in a way that everything begins to normalize when you feel that inner balance. You can keep your blood pressure in check, control your body weight, feel an energy boost, lessen anxiety, banish depression, etc.

5. Improve Health Factors

Another healing effect that you can achieve through qi is the feeling of improvement. When you follow the qi gong methods, after all, you can feel your body's healing process accelerating healing, which is similar to what Reiki practitioners experience. In this case, cultivating qi can mean that minor physical issues will all be gone in time. Eventually, it may even get rid of major concerns that you may have been dealing with for a long time.

6. Treat Different Health Symptoms

While Reiki is similar to qi gong, it has been said that the latter can treat health symptoms. When you experience the qi after the session, you may be able to feel better and banish the symptoms that have plagued your system in the past. You can think of qi gong as the first step towards self-healing on a physical level.

7. Boost Creativity and Intellect

Through qi and the practices associated with it, you will feel it boosting your creativity and intellect. This means that your other activities will also improve because your mind is now ready and fired up for the challenges. You may even find yourself enjoying the tasks, to the point that you find yourself striving to be better than ever.

8. Open Up New Opportunities

When you are practicing qi gong to cultivate your qi, you will be able to open up opportunities to bring it to the next level. After all, qi gong is also used in Chinese martial arts and recreational activities. You will have a chance to manifest the qi that you have cultivated in ways that you have never thought possible. This is just like Reiki healing where you can ascend to different levels.

9. Get Better Sleep

Practicing qi gong and gathering qi within yourself will help you get better sleep. Many have always struggled to sleep, so being able to harness your energy will be a great way to get the sleep that you have always wanted for so long.

10. Feel Joy

Another benefit of getting qi through qi gong is feeling joy. We all go through life with chaos and turmoil all around us, you see. When you practice qi gong, the ideal end result is that you will find happiness and gain the passion and energy that you once had again. Plus, there's something about having joy that genuinely shows its lasting effect will be beneficial for you.

It also helps to know that much of what you learn in Reiki can also be applied and combined with qi gong if you choose to. What matters here is that when you begin to learn how Reiki healing is done in the later chapters, you will feel the energy to get through the day.

What People Have Said After Reiki Sessions

As you journey through the wonders of Reiki, it is nice to know what people have said after their sessions. Their answers vary, but here are the most common responses they have said.

"I feel much better."

This response is common among individuals who have done a Reiki session because there's just nothing like saying that you feel better. With all the negative things going on, the Reiki session really helps to alleviate pain and banish all the negativity from your mind and body. It also comes from the fact that they gain a new kind of energy through the practice.

"I feel more refreshed."

This word of appreciation has been said a lot as people feel tired or exhausted before undergoing the Reiki session. But somehow, after the session, they get the "refreshing" feeling within their body. The reason is that the energy they have been looking for is already inside, and all they need to do is cultivate it through Reiki. It also gives them a new glow that will no doubt be helpful as they continue on with their life.

"I got more focus."

One of the benefits of Reiki is that it gives you more focus. Thus, it is no surprise that this can be something that people will say after a session. By going through Reiki healing, the inner distractions that cloud someone's mind can be banished, so their focus is there all along. They merely have to look deep within, lay on the hands, and concentrate. Then, they will be able to fulfill the goals they have been trying to achieve for so long.

"I can see clearly now."

This statement can mean a lot of things, but this has been said by individuals who have lost their direction. Some of them have merely gone through life without much thought while others have been stressed out with their jobs. But after a few Reiki session, they clearly see what they have to do and go for it without hesitation. Since then, they have never looked back on their decisions or what they truly want in life. Simply put, they have gained a new sense of clarity.

"The pain is gone!"

This is another common thing that you may hear from someone who has done a Reiki session. Whether it is physical or mental, the pain that they have once felt is no longer there. This is also said by folks who have gone to other doctors but still cannot find the treatment that can strip away their pain.

"I get better sleep."

This is one of the benefits that you will get from Reiki healing, so a lot of people who have experienced the practice tend to mention it. For many, sleep is an important part of life, so it can be a bummer when you cannot sleep well after a long day.

After a Reiki session, though, sleep becomes better than ever. It also helps with insomnia and other sleep-related disorders. So, you can say that Reiki healing can give you complete rest.

"I feel calm."

Because Reiki healing helps you banish the negativities that cloud your mind, it brings about calmness and relaxation that can be felt throughout your body. Thus, you feel the universal energy cleanse your body with radiance.

It takes time, but you may find yourself saying one of these statements soon enough, especially when you feel Reiki's wonders.

Chapter 9: How Reiki Can Help Reduce Stress

At the point when a patient comes to me requesting a Reiki treatment, I know they're prepared to discharge old vitality, designs, and/or convictions that no more serve them. They might be completely mindful of this, or simply know on an intuitive level that whatever they've been doing has not been working. The thought of experiencing a Reiki session to adjust their chakras seems to simply feel right.

Reiki is an energy healing strategy that uses "hands-on" and also "hands-off" healing. This strategy can assist in balancing so as to relieve or reducing pain and discomfort the body's vitality focuses, all the more usually known as the chakras. It is a natural process that backings removing so as to relax and healing pieces to the stream of vitality in your body and facilitates adjust and encourage on all levels.

The motivation behind why Reiki can be so capable and successful is on the grounds that it infuses your chakras and your body, with Universal light vitality. Your body takes precisely what it needs to by then. As a practitioner, my responsibility is to just go about as a conduit for Universal vitality keeping in mind the end goal to offer healing brings some support with placing ideally, so that your body can mend itself.

Since Reiki offers us clear vitality some assistance with blocking in our chakras, it is no surprise that a patient feels a great deal more grounded, quiet and loose after a session. A few even sleep during the treatment! Whether alert or napping, Reiki works for the patient's most elevated great.

My practice is in the heart of New York City, an awesome metropolis loaded with opportunities and incitement! For those of us who are overwhelmingly sensitive and effortlessly get on the vitality of others, living in a major city can some of the time overwhelm our sympathetic sensory system? What happens when our sympathetic sensory system is burdened? Our bodies go into battle or-flight mode, and our survival instincts are set into movement.

At the point when this happens, our heart rate increases. We experience shortness of breath, experience issues taking in full breaths, our muscles contract, we might break into a sweat, and our adrenal glands get initiated, therefore shooting up our cortical levels to venture in and offer us some assistance with handling the wellspring of that stress. Adrenaline is our battle or-flight hormone, which also gets enacted by our adrenal glands, and gives us the additional vitality we have to manage (or flee from!) a stressful situation.

Imagine what happens to our bodies when we're in survival mode all the time. Our adrenals get burdened, our adrenals feels shot, we get exhausted, we might hyper-respond, and we might even create physical pains and strains that are not because of physical injury.

This is a reasonable indication that what we've been dealing with enthusiastically has now manifested itself into a physical issue.

In addition, we might assimilate energies that don't fit in with us. This can abandon a few of us feeling irritated, exhausted, drained, and potentially even tired, stressed out and overly on edge.

One of my friend's patients, "L," used to come into my treatment room, often crying with overwhelm when she sat down. It was clear to me that she was all the while working through old examples of self-harm and low self-regard. These examples kept her from enjoying a satisfying adoration life, or from moving forward in her vocation from a verbally injurious supervisor. She was feeling the vitality of everyone around her, since she is a deeply sensitive person. As a result of this she consistently felt off-kilter, scattered, and alarmed, often speaking dangerously fast.

It took her a while to quiet down during her first Reiki treatment. However, before the end of the session I could feel that she had as of now discharged a part of the old energy through her hands and feet, and her chakras were cleared and infused with Universal Light. She shifted to a much more grounded and quiet state, before she even got off the table.

Her eyes were less wild and they shone with I and aliveness, in a way they hadn't some time recently. She was ok with the hush between her words, at the end of the day.

As every session advanced, her inner quality began to rise, and she began to make mindfulness around her self-sabotaging designs. She started to shift them, creating new and more gainful, habits. She began to treat herself with more sympathy and self esteem, began trusting in her intuition, and taking better care of her body, despite her ongoing difficulties.

Things being what they are, how precisely does Reiki delicately and capably bring us back to focus?

Reiki helps us reconnect with our heart, our actual focus, realigning us with our Higher Self.

Apprehension is often a forceful feeling, yet it is eventually a figment, albeit an effective one. Love, however, is genuine. And, Reiki helps us reconnect to ourselves — to Love.

So when we utilize Reiki to get out the vigorous debris in our chakras and reconnect to our self esteem, and in addition our affection for others, we become mindful of the damaging examples we've been holding onto. That is the point at which we can begin to figure out how to break them.

During a Reiki session, you'll feel more settled, and have the capacity to take full, thoughtful and simple breaths. Your muscles begin to discharge pressure, your heart rate will become moderate and adrenals will be comforted. There's a profound sense that everything will be ok, despite the greater part of your battles.

The vast majority benefit from their first Reiki treatment, while others work through more profound issues with additional medications. Everyone's needs are different.

Chapter 10: Increase Your Energy With Reiki

Oddly enough, improvement in your energy levels is actually a side effect of using Reiki. Since Reiki helps you relax and reduce stress, it will automatically increase your natural energy levels. Below is an image of an electromagnetic scan of a human body before and after using Reiki to smooth out the knots and wrinkles in the life force energy. Since it is an electromagnetic field natural to the body, it can be detected and measured with scientific instruments.

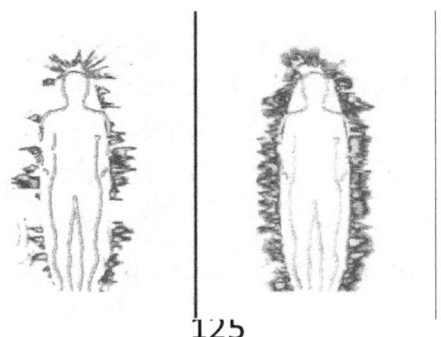

Stress can tear or puncture the energy field running around and through your body. It can also cause blockages. These injuries to your life force energy can cause both acute and chronic conditions to occur that disrupt your general health. The above image shows just how Reiki can help to heal those tears or punctures in that energy field and make it stronger.

The use of Reiki turns off or tones down your body's response to stressors because it takes a large amount of energy to maintain that fight or flight response. If your body is always in a state of agitation, you aren't going to have much energy to devote to anything else, are you?

That fight or flight response is brought about by stimulation of the adrenal glands that sit on top of your kidneys. Adrenaline is a hormone the adrenal glands secrete that gives you a jolt of energy that lets you either fight for your life or the energy to run away. They also secrete cortisol at the same time. Cortisol increases the glucose in the blood since glucose is broken down to provide energy to the muscles.

However, if you have constant secretion of adrenaline and cortisol this can result in higher blood pressure, increased heart rate and high blood glucose levels. If the glucose in your blood isn't made into energy then it is automatically made into fat which is usually deposited in your abdominal region. The increase in fat deposited in your body will increase your weight, which will decrease your energy level and increase the debilitating effects that low energy levels can cause.

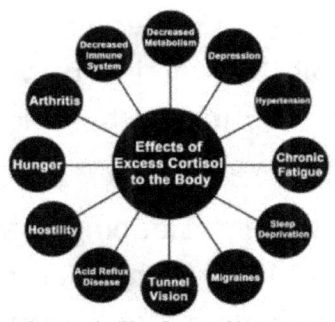

Cortisol - The Stress Hormone

Low energy levels can also make it more difficult for you to sleep, or to stay awake.
I know it sounds confusing but they are actually related. If you are stressed about something, you may not be able to sleep because your mind will go round and round not allowing you to relax enough to sleep. Since you aren't sleeping well, when you wake up you will most likely be tired all day and may find it difficult to remain awake.

The use of Reiki will increase your energy to allow you to fall asleep more easily, sleep deeper and longer, and to awake refreshed. Since you will be sleeping better, you aren't going to find yourself needing that pot of coffee in the morning just to be able to function or wanting to take a power nap just to be able to finish off your shift at work.

Since you will be sleeping better and having a higher level of that natural energy flowing through your body, you will find that you can think more clearly and make more rational decisions. That mental clarity can make you less mentally exhausted since you won't have to work as hard to piece thoughts together.

Now, I know that I have talked a lot about how Reiki can help you and about Reiki therapists and sessions. But what if the budget is tighter than a cork stuck in a bottle? Well, relax! Yes, that pun was intended. You don't have to shell out a lot of money to get the benefits of Reiki. Like I said before, anyone can learn Reiki. Even you.

Chapter 11: The Signs

Usui saw the signs show up to him when he was on a spiritual pursuit in a bubble of light. These signs are made use of in the technique of Buddhism to which he was additionally a specialist of.

When one gets to the 2nd degree of Reiki as well as the Master degree have access to is offered to the specialist of spiritual signs and also words. They boost the circulation of life power reliant after the sign being made use of.

Others think that each sign has its very own awareness and also could be moderated after to get magnificent info on just how to make use of each sign. The Reiki procedure in fact equips the signs so they could accomplish their designated objectives.

The signs offer as power sets off like a response in the human physical body to stimulation. There are those Mystical Buddhist sects that think all signs stand for some concept of Buddhism reveal as well as ought to be secret and also spiritual for that factor. They will certainly additionally claim that all composing in recommendation to spiritual concerns is spiritual and also any person being revealed the writing will certainly experience the sign being dental implanted as a seed in their importance.

Sign 5.

Raku.

(obvious Ra Koo).

Pen name:: Grounding as well as Closing.

This is the conclusion sign in a Reiki session.

Its function it to ground the individual that obtained the therapy. It works in the recovery of the Kundalini, hara link and also.

The Raku sign is utilized in the last stage of an attunement. The striking lightning screw sign is attracted downwards from paradise to planet.

The number 11 is missing out on in the image over considering that some individuals error the number 11 as component of the sign. This is sign is superb to make use of where practical is not feasible.

This is a far-off recovery sign that is made use of over both range and also time (previously, existing and also future) to recover anything or any person. It is additionally sent out in range attunement.

Hon: Spirit, Resource, Beginning, Universe.

Sha: Mind, Making it through.

Ze: Area, Be, Being.

Sho: Sensations Feelings.

Nen: Conscious, Physical body, Interest.

This sign is made use of for recovery over a big range; in case the client isn't really in the visibility of the therapist. You could send this sign throughout an area, throughout the road, throughout community, to various other components of the nation and also globe.

You could send this sign right into the future like a battery to save to be accessed when required. This 3rd sign likewise offers as a secret that opens the Akashic Records. For this factor this sign is made use of to recover the internal youngster as well as previous lives.

This sign likewise has a message that the Buddha in me is there to welcome the Buddha in you. It is when the link is stated and also recognized via our hearts that you are the recipient of a state of Divine Union and also Reiki could be discussed no matter of the range.

This sign could likewise be utilized to recover karmic patterns and also propensities we have that show as illness or psychological or psychological discomfort as well as distress as a result of its relationship to the Akashic Records.

Various educators could attract the signs in different ways to pass on the sign yet that does not alter the power made use of in Reiki for recovery. Some individuals completely finish up counting just on the signs and also finish up venerating the signs as resisted to comprehending their partnership to the global power pressure. For some the signs do it and also others require sound called Kotodama as well as intents to conjure up the power for themselves.

The names of the signs that are utilized largely in the west are made use of as Concepts to materialize the power. When a Reiki master reveals his pupil the signs he is making a perception on the pupils mind that links with esoteric power that the sign stands for. Since the sign comes to be a component of the professional every time the specialist attracts, states or creates the sign the power is conjured up from that sign.

Bringing the Reiki Symbols right into being could be acted of methods. They could be:.

- Stating the signs name repeatedly like a concept.

- Leading to the signs name 3 times.

- Attracting them with your finger.

- Attracting them with your hand.

- Traced airborne.

- Attracting them with your 3rd eye.

- Some individuals also attract the signs on paper as they function, this is not the conventional means however if it functions its all great.

You use the sign or signs in your hands/ hands revising them or re imagining them on the customer. Usage whatever technique you desire remember that intent is necessary.

Sign 2.

Sei Hei Ki.

(Pronounced Claim Hay Trick).

Psychological Psychological Indication.

Pen name: Mental/Emotional Sign.

Definition: "God and also Male Upcoming With each other".

or.

"Trick To Deep space".

It is made use of for Psychological Recovery; Psychological Healing/Emotional Recovery as well as Relaxing the Mind.

Sei: I Direct.

Hei: The Bow/Arrow To.

Ki: Vital force, Light, Recognition.

This sign functions with the reason of illness that is typically concealed in the subconscious mind, which is the psychological mind, or the aware mind as a psychological physical body. This sign stands for the equilibrium in between the right as well as left side of the human brain. This sign is utilized in recovery people with anxiety, dependencies, rage and also connection problems.

Objective: This sign deals with the subconscious to promote psychological as well as psychological recovery along with to help in self-programming with problems of obsession and also points of that nature. Some instructors utilize it on the very first 4 Chakras just and also some utilize it on all. This Sign assists to stabilize the right as well as left sides of the human brain in order for recovery both undesirable routines as well as computer programming in wanted routines.

Purpose: The intension in this sign is consistency. It could additionally be utilized to detoxify a space, food, water complied with by the initial sign. It is additionally recognized as the "Love" sign and also the sign standing for the Buddha.

The major usages of this sign are for:.

psychological as well as psychological recovery.

Psychic Security.

Purifying.

In arbitrations to trigger the Kundalini.

To Stabilize the right and also left sides of the Human brain.

Help in healing/removing dependencies.

Recovering previous injuries.

Removes psychological clog as well as lines up the top chakras.

Eliminates both unfavorable and also bad resonances.

Recovers psychological equilibrium as well as consistency.

Dia Ko Myo.

(Pronounced Dye Ko Me O).

Pen name:" Master Sign".

This is the sign of the Reiki Master.

All the Reiki Embodies is show in this sign. It is the sign of the 3rd degree or Master. With Reiki it improves both psychic and also instinct that one has.

1. You begin with the very first Reiki sign Cho Ku Rei or the sign of the physical body. This books the power to the factor on the recipient via the professional's hands.

You after that focus on the 2nd Reiki Sign Sei He Ki to advertise filtration and also purifying. This sign is likewise utilized to remove the customer of contaminants and also illness.

The 3rd sign is utilized for those Receivers of Reiki that could not be touched. This is utilized mostly in range recovery.

4. Tan A Ra Sha is after that utilized to ground and also unblock any kind of power circulation. It could likewise currently be utilized to minimize any kind of discomfort in the recipient.

* This is the sign of the Reiki Master. The 4th sign Dia Ko Myo remarks on the partnership in between humankind, the universe and also Reiki.

Others think that each sign has its very own awareness and also could be moderated after to get magnificent info on exactly how to utilize each sign. Various instructors might attract the signs in different ways to pass on the sign yet that does not transform the power utilized in Reiki for recovery. Due to the fact that the sign ends up being a component of the specialist every time the professional attracts, claims or creates the sign the power is conjured up from that sign. It is likewise understood as the "Love" sign and also the sign standing for the Buddha.

You begin with the initial Reiki sign Cho Ku Rei or the sign of the physical body.

The very first 3 signs are made use of in combination to every various other to match the demands ideal of the customer.

Cho Ku Rei as well as She He Ki are utilized with each other to clean the physique of points like contaminants as well as conditions; while Cho Ku Rei as well as Hon Sha Ze Sho Nen could be made use of with each other to advertise recovery at a range.

The Meridians could come to be obstructed go stale or circulation in the incorrect instructions creating disease and also psychological inequality. When Qi/Ki could not move in the physical body, we could not have optimal health and wellness or equilibrium in our physical beings, which influences our souls.

The Meridians are 12 power courses in the physical body that Qi/Ki streams via. These are clear power courses in the human physical body that promote power. Each meridian matches to a physical body feature as well as or body organ.

With Reiki the life pressure is funnelled via the Chakra right into the physical body.

Power takes a trip with the Nadis (blood vessels in Sanskrit) and also Meridians which are a network of psychic nerves or rising as well as coming down spiral power.

The 7 major Chakras are linked by 3 significant nadis which parallel one an additional. These associate to our activities as well as preparing, to physical as well as psychological task and also the feeling that we are people, different from the various other. It is the power activity of the nadis that influenced the sign that is utilized in medication called the caduceus.

The level of chakra and also meridian task is reliant on an individual's state of wellness and also being. If a chakra is ruined or obstructed it will certainly restrain the circulation of Qi/Ki in the physical body along the meridians resulting in inequalities. In basic, the front face of a chakra associates to our psychological features as well as the backs our wills to work.

The Chakras Separately

1. Origin chakra (connected shade: red; associated components of the physical body: adrenal glandulars, kidneys, spine, leg bones).

The origin chakra premises us in physical presence (our physical bodies and also the worldly globe). Well balanced origin chakras lead to a healthy and balanced need for the essentials of life (food, heat, sanctuary, and so on) When this chakra is unbalanced, we might hesitate of life, take out from physical fact, really feel taken advantage of, run in a very egocentric method, or lean to physical violence. Disorder of this chakra additionally could cause issues of the feet, legs and also reduced back.

Equally as the Meridians associate to a physical body component so does the Chakras.

Along with the Physical body's 7 Key Chakras there are regarding 122 small one's. The physical body's several small chakras (there go to the very least 122) like sets behind the eyes, near the ears, behind the knees, as well as on the soles of the feet and also hands of the hands. Anywhere there is a joint; there is a chakra, so the hands have numerous power.

The hand chakras are the ones where Reiki recovery power is routed. As soon as a master educator attunes you to the resource of Reiki, objective is all that is needed for you to funnel this power. It streams right into your physical body with your crown and also heart chakras as well as out via your hand chakras to any place you route it (to certain components of your physical body or to others).

Each significant chakra on the front of the physical body is coupled with its equivalent on the back. With each other they are thought about to be the front as well as back element of one chakra. The origin and also crown chakras could be thought about paired since they are the flexible factors of the physical body's major power existing, which raises and also down the back and also right into which every one of the chakras factor

The suggestion is to stabilize the power just as in each chakra so the recipient in turn will certainly really feel well balanced both literally, psychologically, mentally and also emotionally. As a Reiki session startings, the chakras are removed. When the Chakra is well balanced and also stimulated effectively the power degree increases standing for spiritual enjoyable.

Right here is a listing of the chakras of the physique:

The chakras and also the physique

Every chakra has a matching body organ in our physical system

The origin chakra belongs along with the big bowel as well as the anus. It likewise has a particular impact on the feature of the kidneys.

The navel chakra comes from the recreation system, the testicles as well as ovaries and the urinary bladder and also kidneys.

The solar plexus chakra remains in relationship to the liver, gall bladder, belly, spleen and also the tiny gut.

The heart chakra comes from the heart and also the arms.

The throat chakra associates with the lungs as well as the throat.

The 3rd eye (temple) chakra comes from the human brain, face, nose, eyes and so on

. Royalty chakra does not have an equivalent body organ yet belongs to the entire being.

There is a clear link in between the problem of a chakra as well as the problem of the matching body organ. A chakra could be over energetic, under energetic or in equilibrium. Making use of

Reiki could offer the chakras equilibrium as well as the body organs wellness.

Chakras and also the endocrine system.

The chakras transform power from one degree to an additional by dispersing Ki (additionally called Chi, Prana, Mana depending on idea system) to the physical body. According to practice, each chakra additionally matches to one of the significant glandulars in the physical body.

The origin chakra remains in connection to the adrenal glandular.

The navel chakra to the ovaries or testicles.

The solar plexus chakra is associated with the pancreatic.

The heart chakra belongs along with the thymus.

The throat chakra represents the thyroid glandular.

The 3rd eye chakra has a link to the pituitary glandular.

Royalty chakra is typically attached to the pineal glandular.

The endocrine system plays a significant part for the physical body's day-to-day wellness. The glandulars launch bodily hormones straight right into the blood stream as well as control all facets of development, growth as well as everyday tasks.

Physical issues are typically the outcome of an obstruction in the power circulation in the system comprised of meridians and also chakras triggering the body organs or glandulars to not work appropriately.

Chapter 12: Symbols Of Reiki

You might be aware of a Reiki session from a self-practiced session, or you might just hear about it. Reiki is an ancient healing method based on the energy transformation in the body. It is a great mental, physical, and emotional healing process, which has an amazing amount of health benefits.

The most amazing and significant features of Reiki are its symbols. These symbols allow people to continue their healing sessions and experience the energy of the universe. In most of the cases, the symbols only affect the involuntary actions of the body. However, the Reiki symbols work in a different method. These symbols change and modify the functioning of mind and body. The Reiki practitioners envision of Reiki's symbols and loudly say their names draw them in the healing process. If you are utilizing your intentions in the initiation process, then you will experience success for your efforts.

Therefore, it is significant to know about the symbols of Reiki and their actual meaning. These symbols have always been kept in secret; however, the research and exposure in the past few years influenced the symbols, and we have collected quite a lot of information. Here is the most important information regarding Reiki's symbols.

1. The Power Symbol: Cho Ku Rei

The powerful symbol of Cho Ku Rei is utilized to boost or reduce the power depending on the specific direction. The purpose of this symbol is to illuminate the light switch, which represents its capability to brighten up our spirituality. It is quite similar to the coil, which is believed by Reiki practitioners to increase and limit the energy flow in the human body. The power could be in different forms in Cho Ku Rei. This symbol is highly effective in the physical healing and purification of the soul. It can also be utilized in drawing attention and the focus of an individual.

If you are thinking to enhance or decrease your power, then Cho Ku Rei is the perfect symbol for you. It can be recognized by portraying a coil, which can be in clockwise or counterclockwise, representing chi that is the movement of energy from the body. You can think about a switch for imagining the power symbol. When this switch is activated or on, then a Reiki practitioner has a higher capability to brighten up the energy channel in your body.

Effectively Utilization of Cho Ku Rei

Cho Ku Rei is normally utilized at the beginning of a Reiki session. It assists in enhancing energy and power at any point in the ongoing session. One of the most common ways of utilizing Cho Ku Rei is while healing a wound or injury. It can be highly effective in dealing with common to severe pains or injuries.

In theoretical terms, Cho Ku Rei can be great in clearing out negative thoughts, energy, and feelings from your body that could be an obstacle in your Reiki session. If you are dealing with negative energy in your body, then Cho Ku Rei is the solution to your problems. It helps in taking the symbols out of your body and assist in filling it with light and positivity.

Cho Ku rei can be highly beneficial in improving the strength of your relationships. Moreover, Cho Ku Rei can be effective in getting a job or working on getting a job or relationship with your loved ones. It can also provide protection against different misfortunes, which happens because of having unclean energy in the body. Therefore, utilizing Cho Ku Rei could be a great boost in improving your energy system. On the other hand, if you are thinking to give a natural advancement in your nutrition, then Cho Ku Rei is the solution for removing negativity from your food and system.

2. The Harmony Symbol: Sei he ki

This symbol represents harmony. The primary purpose of this symbol is purification for improving the mental and emotional healing process. This symbol is identical to the beach wave, which has the natural capability of washing and sweeping negative feelings. Different Reiki practitioners utilize this symbol while treating patients of depression and addiction. It helps in improving the natural balanced state of the body. It can also help treat the patients to recover from the emotional or physical state of disturbance. The symbol of Sei he ki is highly important in unblocking the creative energies of our system.

If you have been looking to purify and balance your emotional and mental health, then sei he ki is the perfect solution for you. The symbol of sei he ki is quite similar to a wave getting ready to crash the bird's wing or the beach. The symbol is extremely beneficial in establishing a balanced state between right and left-brain. It also serves as the protection symbol. You need to establish a healthy balance in your brain to perform your daily tasks in a perfect manner.

Effective Utilization of sei he ki

Have you been looking to remember new information for taking a test or improving your memory? Then sei he ki is the perfect solution for you. You can draw a symbol of sei he ki on your book during reading or studying for improving your memorizing power. You will remember the information for years. If you just utilize this symbol of Reiki during visualization, you will experience a boost in your information.

Moreover, if you have been struggling to quit some habits like drinking or smoking, then turning to see he ki could be highly beneficial for you. Remember, people adopt bad habits after experiencing some bad energy. If you utilize the symbol of sei he ki around you, then you can reduce negativity and spread positivity to get rid of bad habits.

Having headaches could be another form of dealing with depression or poor mental and emotional health. You can consult sei he ki for getting rid of your headaches as well. You can eliminate your headaches and the habit of consuming different unnecessary medications. Sei he ki also helps in giving you protection from negativity. This symbol removes negative from your body. Even better, it can enhance your positive affirmations. If you write affirmations daily, then try drawing sei he ki next to them. You will experience great positive and motivational energy within your body.

3. The Distance Symbol: Hon sha ze sho nen

This symbol is highly effective in sending qi over large distance locations. The intention of this symbol is timelessness. It contains a tower-like appearance, which provides the basis of its second name as a pagoda. The primary function of this symbol is to bring people together over different time or space. Hon sha ze sho nen can change itself for unchaining the Akashic records, which is believed to be the fundamental source of human awareness. Reiki practitioners consider this an ideal tool in dealing with previous life issues and inner-child state of customers.

The idea of hon sha ze sho nen is a little difficult to understand as compared to other symbols of Reiki. The primary meaning of hon sha ze sho nen is having no present, past, or future. This symbol is utilized for sending energy and power of Reiki in different space and time. Moreover, this symbol cannot change your past; however, it provides healing to deal with past traumatic situations.

It can help in the identification of actual life experiences and getting over old wounds and injuries. The symbol of hon sha ze sho nen can help to turn an awful incident into a learning experience. The symbol helps Reiki practitioners to send the energy in the future that could result in some bad news of exams, jobs, or tough communication with our special loved ones.

Effective utilization of hon sha ze sho nen

Hon sha ze sho nen is a little different than utilizing the other symbols of Reiki. Hon sha ze sho nen is one of the most powerful symbols of Reiki; however, correct implementation is required for getting results. This symbol works effectively on the subtle body than that of a physical body. Therefore, Reiki practitioners recommend utilizing this symbol regularly for successful healing of past, present, and future.

4. The Master Symbol: Dai ko myo

This symbol represents the whole concept of Reiki. The primary purpose of this symbol is to bring enlightenment to the body. Reiki masters only use this symbol while initiating the attunement. This symbol allows healing by bringing the power of healing. It is one of the most complicated forms of symbols to be drawn with hands during a Reiki session.

All power to the wonderful symbol of daily ko myo, which is also the master symbol. This is responsible for bringing nourishment and enlightenment to the body. Therefore, this is also known as the holiest symbol of Reiki. It brings the great forces of vibration and provides the awesome transformational power than all the other five symbols of Reiki. The healing powers of dai ko myo consist of the upper chakra by involving the soul in general. Dai ko myo is the representation of empowerment and represents the meaning of 'bringing shining light' in the body. This process of spiritual empowerment through dai ko myo helps in getting closer to God with the help of Reiki practitioners.

Utilization of Dai ko myo

You can utilize different methods to visualize, think, and draw the symbol of dai ko myo for getting it to your third eye. You can meditate with dai ko myo for receiving and nourishing your soul or body. It releases amazing power to help yourself and the world.

On the other hand, if you are thinking to improve your relationship and establish awareness to get better spiritual insight, then dai ko myo is the most significant symbol for you. Utilizing this symbol along with other symbols of Reiki can do wonders for you. Dai ko myo is an excellent way of improving the health of your immune system. Dai ko myo helps in improving the energy flow in your body. It helps in removing blocked particles that could be affecting your immune system. If you are taking any homeopathic medications to improve your health, then considering dai ko myo could enhance your capability to avail from the benefits and improving your well-being.

5. The Completion Symbol: Raku

This symbol is utilized during the last stages of the Reiki session. Grounding is the primary purpose of this symbol. The Reiki practitioners turn to this symbol during the end of a Reiki session. They utilize this symbol for closing, settling, and sealing the qi within the human body. The outstanding lightning bolt is the ideal symbol, which is drawn by the hand movement during the completion of the Reiki session.

Raku is an ideal symbol of Reiki, which can be utilized at the master level. Raku symbol is also known as fire serpent; however, just having a look at its shape will tell you the reason for its name. It contains a zigzag bolt-like shape that is greatly utilized for grounding a Reiki session. It is similar to the utilization of savasana at the end of a yoga session, which helps the body to absorb and get all the advantages of Reiki. This symbol is effective in clearing and removing any negative energy from the body during the practice.

Utilization of Reku

It is highly effective to utilize the symbol of Reku at the end of the Reiki session for getting all the energy and benefits of the process. You can draw the symbol for experiencing the grounding benefits in daily life.

Utilizing Multiple Reiki Symbols at the Same Time

You do not need to utilize these symbols individually; however, they can be utilized in combination with other symbols at the same time. One of the significant ways of doing this is by sending Reiki's energy for treating a sick child. You can hold the picture of the child and start visualizing Cho Ku Rei, sei her ki, hon sha ze sho nen, and Cho Ku Rei with three repetitions per symbol. You can call recipient name three times by holding his or her picture in your hand; this could be a great way of sending healing energies to them.

You can utilize these symbols for curing a future event with the help of Reiki. It could be bad news, a job interview, a marriage proposal, or a doctor's appointment. You can simply repeat Cho Ku Rei, sei he ki, hon sha ze sho nen, and Cho Ku Rei with three repetitions. This will bring you peace, relaxation, and positive energy to help you deal with that day. You will lose feelings of depression, anxiety, and stress with the help of Reiki. You will focus on building positivity around you.

These symbols are an amazing way of enhancing your mental, spiritual, emotional, and physical health. If you have never received a Reiki session, then you should give one try to it. Reiki will assist you in understanding these symbols and signs more effectively to improve your daily life.

Chapter 13: Reiki Section

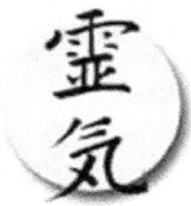

1.1 The History and Origin of Reiki

The origin of Reiki can be traced back as far back as the ancient Tibet, in the late 1800 by Dr. Mikao Usui of Japan.

Unfortunately back in the old days Reiki Traditions were taught orally, which mean that the information was passed on from masters to student by word of mouth.

Throughout the years, the Reiki story has been embellished by storyteller. We don't know for sure which story is true, but what we do know to be true is that Mikao Usui rediscovered Reiki while on Mount

Kurama on a 21-day retreat to fast and meditate.

After his revelation Mikao Usui practiced Reiki for a few years on his own, then he started teaching it to others. The first Reiki Master he taught Reiki to was Chijuro Hayashi, who developed with the help of Mikao Usui the basic hands position we now use when we do Reiki.

Chijuro Hayashi later Taught Hawayo Takata whose origins were in Japan, but who lived in Hawaii. She brought Reiki to the Western part of the world. Before her death, Hawayo Takata taught Reiki to her grand daughter Phyllis Lei Furumote and 22 other Reiki Master.

1.2 Reiki PreceptsJust for today only:

☐Do not anger.

☐Do not worry.

☐Be humble.

☐Do your work honestly.

☐Be compassionate to all living being.

Mikao Usui, founder of the system of Reiki, believed the precepts to be important guides to spiritual development and healing. Finding ways to connect with them in daily life is a great way to support one's inner growth.

1.3 What is Reiki?

Reiki is considered by some people as a natural or holistic therapy. Some people describe it as a path of self development and transformation.

It is also said that: Reiki is a therapy that allows any stagnant and blocked energy found within the physical body or in the energy field surrounding the body to be released.

Although Reiki is said to be simple yet powerful technique that everyone can learn. Reiki is a wonderful gift of love to receive and to offer. Reiki energy is pure unconditional love that you can safely share with your family, friends and pet.

Reiki is non invasive and is an excellent complementary therapy that can safely be used with any other form of therapy.

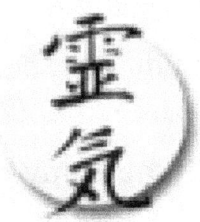

1.4 What is Reiki for Animals?

Reiki for animals is basically the same as Reiki for humans. The only differences that are found in the practice of Reiki for Animals is the way you communicate and get information from the animal.

Because animals don't communicate the same with the Reiki Therapist as a human would, the therapist as to rely on his or her intuitive ability to communicate and be receptive to the information given by the pet and found in its energy.

1.5 Who can become a Reiki Animal Healer?

Everyone who has been attuned by a certified Reiki Master, and who the desire to become a Reiki Animal Healer can!

1.6 Which animal can benefit from receiving a Reiki treatment?

All animal, without any exception can benefit from a Reiki treatment.

1.7 Meaning of the word Reiki

The word « REIKI », consiste of 2 Japanese syllables, which once put together from a word that means: Universal life energy.

Reï : Energy

Ki :Universal life

1.8 What will Reiki do for your animal?

Reiki will help your pet release any stagnant or blocked energy that maybe causing your pet dis-comfort or dis-ease. Reiki helps pets regenerate and recuperate their vitality. Reiki helps your pet heal faster after surgery, during or after an illness. Reiki helps pets who have been rescued to feel safe and loved once again. Reiki can be used to help your pet's crossover when they are approaching the transition from life to after life. Reiki can also be used to release any side effects from medication, boost the energy level in the water they drink and bathe in and Reiki can even be used to boost the vitamin and protein in your pet's food.

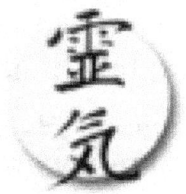

1.9 Here are the main benefits of a Reiki Animal Healing Treatment: One of the greatest Reiki healing health benefits is stress reduction and relaxation, which triggers the body's natural healing abilities, and help maintain good health. Reiki healing is a natural therapy that gently balances life energies and brings health and well being to the recipient.

This simple, non-invasive healing system works with the Higher Self of the Receiver to promote health and well being of the entire physical, emotional and psychic body. Therefore it is truly a healing therapy which promotes wholeness of the Mind, Body and Soul.

1.10 What happens during a Reiki healing session?

The Reiki practitioner prepare themselves, they way they were taught after they were attuned to Reiki, and proceed by channeling the chi energy and redistribute this soothing, loving and healing energy within the animals body and energy field.

When necessary the Reiki practitioner will cleanse, and release any negative energy that is found and that maybe jeopardizing the animal's health and wellbeing, then he will replace that energy with more rejuvenating energy that will allow the animal to feel balance, calm, and centered.

Reiki treatment can be given directly to some animal by laying the practitioners hands directly or right above the animal's chakras. In some case, the practitioner, for safety reason, will find it easier to send Reiki Love and Light energy via a distant healing technique taught to them in their Reiki attunement workshop.

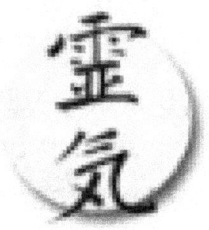

1.11 Can a Reiki help my pet when it is time for it to crossover?

Yes Reiki can help your pet crossover. I know that we all love our pets. I also know that this subject is a very sensitive subject, because we all wish we could keep our pets with us for ever and ever.

When the time comes that we have to let go of our pets, Reiki can help not only the pet but also the human companion during the transition. Reiki will provide comfort and soothing energy for our animals and to ourselves.

Reiki can be used to help sooth the physical and emotional pain that our pet maybe experimenting due to the dis-ease or the fear of leaving their human companion behind.

Reiki will surround your pets with love and light, thus making the transition easier on the pet and its human companion. Reiki will give everyone involved in the process a sense of deep love and sooth everyone's grief.

Remember: Reiki treatments comfort the mind, body and spirit, leaving the animal feeling relaxed and peaceful, but can never be used to replace a veterinarian's care.

1.12 How does Reiki energy work?

The animals and every other living thing in this universe are made from energy. With the use of hands on healing technique that Reiki teaches, you are able to treat the energy within the animal's body and around it.

You will find seven main chakras within the animal's body. The chakras are all perfectly aligned with the animal's spine. (Chakras are located from the top of head to the base of the spine). These chakras and their functions will be revealed to you, a little later in the book.

Each chakra has specific functions, when they are in harmony with one another, the animal is healthy, he is full of energy and loving life, but if there is an energy blockage, stagnant energy or negative energy accumulated within the chakras or in the energy field. The animal often suffers from: anxiety, irritability, hyper activeness, fatigue, dis-comfort and even disease.

With the help of specific hands-on or hands-free technique the Reiki Therapist is able to assist the animal, in releasing the unwanted energy. Rebalancing and harmonizing the pet's energy back a normal adequate energy flow.

Chapter 14: Harnessing The Power Of Reiki

Anyone who has been exposed to Reiki energies through treatments that they receive from others will normally feel the urge to learn and practice Reiki himself or herself. This is not just a great addition to your own life but is also a wonderful way to help the people around you. Harnessing the true power of Reiki can help you take good care of yourself. For many, this is a life- transforming experience that can improve the quality of life and also the goals and aims that you set for yourself.

Reiki allows you to address the needs of your soul, body and mind. Conscious living comes with the constant practice of Reiki. It restores your body to its ability function at its best by slowly guiding you towards what your body requires. Your own potential for healing naturally increases as you are completely in tune with yourself when you practice Reiki. Now, there is great power in an individual that can actually help you manifest anything you desire, be it physical health, mental health or even your goals.

Harnessing the power of Reiki to manifest thoughts and ideas: We have all witnessed people who seem to have everything going for them in their lives. These are the people who are able to set their mind on a certain goal and just achieve them with great ease. Then there are people who try and try and still seem like they never get their due. The question is the former just lucky? Or is there some secret to their consistent success?

Unknown to most of us lays some power that is always active. This power exists just outside our conscious being. It is very easy to access and can be operated by all of us with the practice of Reiki. Philosophers and practitioners of Reiki call this the power of manifestation. It is created by the mind and is available to every individual. When you are able to communicate with the Universe constantly, this power can be harnessed quite easily.

For most of us, it seems like this power of manifestation is just unavailable because we do not pay attention to your own thoughts. There is constant inner dialogue that we are distracted from for the most part. If you have heard of saints and prophets who are able to perform miracles with the power of their mind, you are probably hearing the stories of people whose souls are advanced enough to harness this power of manifestation.

We all have dreams and desires that we either express or keep within ourselves. When our wishes are half-hearted, we are unable to generate enough energy to manifest these thoughts into reality. The attention that we pay to the obstacles standing between our goals and us makes this even worse and just pushes us further and further away from the life that we could be living.

Different planes of manifestation: Manifesting your thoughts into reality takes a fixed path always. There are different planes that this process takes until you actually see your idea or goal as reality.

The Causal plane: The moment you have a thought or an idea, you enter the causal plane. This is almost like a spark that ignites the process of manifestation. So, when you look at something and wish that you had it for yourself, you have begun your journey on the path of manifestation.

The Mental plane: Now that you have an idea, you are bound to think about it. When you enter this stage that makes you actively think about ways to make your idea a reality you enter the mental plane. The idea is now turning into a thought. Your job is to give some structure to this thought by giving it more details. It is recommended that you do this in the written form. Make step-by-step plans and even add drawings if you are able to. The more details you add to your plan, the closer you will get to your goal. When you have the final written structure for your goals, it is known as the "convincer." It is very important to give your goals structure as though they have already been achieved. Now that your ideas are concrete, you need to provide them with the energy that they need to become a reality. This happens in the next plane.

The Astral plane: When you begin to give your ideas and thoughts positive energies, you begin to enter the Astral or Emotional plane. You can do this by giving Reiki to the structure that you have created. The moment your thoughts get the positive energy that they need, they will manifest themselves in the final plane, which is the Physical Plane.

This is the path that is followed by manifestation regardless of what you want to achieve. Whether it is good health, money or even peaceful relationships, you just need that idea or spark that will set the energies going. Then, with Reiki you are able to harness this power and catalyze the process of manifestation.

Giving Reiki to your thoughts

The first thing to do when you enter the Mental Plane of an idea or thought is to understand how much of your focus is on the goal itself. Most often, we tend to focus on the problems. This may include the problem that is getting in the way of achieving the goal or the problems that we trying to eliminate by accomplishing the goal. Focusing on either problem reduces the power of your positive thoughts. You are likely to send out the problems as the message to the Universe. Make sure that all your thoughts are focused on the goal. That is when your emotional energy begins to get aligned.

As soon as this emotional energy is aligned with the energy that your goal requires, relax and keep the focus. Trust the universe to help you achieve the goals that you have set for yourself. If you are a Reiki I practitioner, giving about 15 minutes of Reiki to your convincer will energize the goal. For those who are practicing level II or above, you have several more options. You have the ability to use the absent treatment symbol and then provide energy through communications channels using the emotional or mental techniques. This accelerates the process of manifestation. You can learn these techniques and practice meditation consistently to harness the complete power of your Reiki.

When you have provided Reiki to your goals, do not think about it too much. Just send it back into your Universe and release it completely. This can be hard for most people to do. However, if you try consciously, you will be able to get your mind off the goal completely. Being attached to anything, even your goal will help you harness the power of Reiki completely. End your day by giving thanks always, whether you have achieved the goal or not.

The moment your goal has been manifested in the Physical plane, it is absolutely necessary to send thanks to the universe, your spirit guides and the gods and goddesses of your belief. Gratitude is one of the most essential things to make your Reiki work to its full capacity.

With this simple process, you will see that nothing is impossible or beyond you. When you are able to harness and release Reiki, you have the power to manifest just about anything.

Chapter 15: Reiki Healing Success Sories

SOPHIE AND REIKI SELF-CARE

Sophie used Reiki's treatment to help with pain, surgical recovery and general well-being Sophie could never have known Reiki unless she was living next door to a Reiki master. She wanted to be a good neighbor and she accepted an invitation to participate in the Reiki intro program.

Sophie was on more medicines than she liked, and she was around 80 years of age. She worried about the increased pain in her joints and feared a future operation. Sophie was convinced to learn that Reiki helps with pain, allowing many patients (under their physicians ' supervision) to minimize or avoid their pain medications. And since Reiki therapy strengthens the body's natural healing ability, it makes sense that it can help individuals get up and faster after surgery. She signed up for the next class, feeling she had little to lose.

Sophie found her Reiki class to admire and particularly enjoyed the emphasis on health rather than illness. Reiki was a soothing surprise, unlike anything she had done before. Even after the first class session, harmony persisted and engulfed her again when she studied at home. Back in class, Sophie felt hesitant at first when she practiced together with her classmates to position her Reiki hands, but her self-awareness quickly melts away.

While Reiki was repeatedly told by the teacher that she was primarily self-handling, Sophie saw the familiar feeling in her hands as she cuddled her grandson before her bed and was shocked when the usually stubborn boy slept on her lap. She told her friends frequently, "I have in my hands a treasure." Sophie, she took her treasure into surgery, giving herself Reiki even while she was waiting on the gurney. As she was aware in the recovery room, she put her Reiki hands comfortably in her abdomen or chest and noticed that the incision had soothed Reiki's pain. She continued to give herself Reiki several times a day after recovery. Sophie was released a day earlier than expected from the hospital.

Five years later, Sophie is doing Reiki every day. She and two Reiki friends come to share treatment every week— they call it their "Reiki bee "— and she is pleased that she sometimes requests a Reiki session from their daughter.

Sophie and her doctor had some drugs stopped and others through. He believes Reiki is likely why he doesn't get distracted by the side effects that she still wants. "I always knew that it makes sense to be a good neighbor," she says, "but I never thought my life could change!"

HOW SUSAN GOT REIKI TO SUPPORT WITH FATIGUE

Susan was a pediatric nurse for the last 20 years. She loved taking care of children, but had to admit lately that tiredness slipped into her days and stopped her from spending time away from the hospital. Previously, two of her nurse colleagues had studied Reiki and wanted to give her a session. Sophie did not know why she felt so nervous, but she decided to accept her call when nothing else eased this constant tiredness.

One Friday night, her colleagues came home to give her Reiki. They told her to sleep until the next day she woke up by herself. After 12 hours of deep sleep she could recall, there wasn't much left in the night. Susan was seeing something next week that made her think seriously about learning how to practice Reiki herself. Caroline called her friends and said, "It is like my body forgot to sleep well and the Reiki remembered it." A boy with sickle cell anemia was screaming and writhing, with intense pain and often no reaction to medication. Her colleagues put their hands on the boy, and he slept peacefully, his body fully relaxed, within five minutes.

HOW CAROLINE WAS ASSISTED BY REIKI DURING BREAST CANCER TREATMENT

No time to diagnose breast cancer is easy, but it is especially difficult to diagnose Caroline. Her husband was sent to Madrid for a special mission and she looked forward to the time abroad and a chance to mold her Spanish. The timing of her trip now coincided with the time of her treatment for cancer. As her diagnosis in Spain could not be completed, Caroline decided to travel. Then search for additional assistance.

Caroline was practical enough to know that she needed many levels of support. She wanted emotional support to relieve the medical symptoms and the depression her day and night had. Caroline's doctor warned that many people found the treatment to be exhausting, and Caroline would add to it with frequent flying tiredness. She was interested in pain and, given her history of pharmaceutical sensitivity, she was sure she would experience other side effects of treatment.

Fortunately, her counseling facility had a Reiki system. Caroline paired Reiki with each visit to the doctor and chemotherapy session. Because even on a good day she became susceptible to anxiety, she wanted to receive Reiki before her chemo. She found that getting Reiki reduced her depression, but also her discomfort at first considerably.

Caroline weathered and completed her diagnosis on schedule. Once at home, Caroline continued to receive Reiki privately monthly. Eventually she began to practice Reiki as a means of protecting her health and controlling her addiction to anxiety.

Chapter 16: Reiki And Aromatherapy

Although Reiki is very powerful (yet subtle), practitioners say that adding in other forms of energy healing enhances the session for both patient and practitioner. One such alternative modality often added to Reiki sessions is aromatherapy. Aromatherapy is defined as healing through scent, which improves physical, mental, and emotional well-being.

Aromatherapy basics

Essential oils are naturally occurring volatile fragrant compounds that are found in parts of plants like the seeds, stems, bark, roots, flowers. Aromatherapy is a holistic healing method that incorporates essential oils for health and well-being. Aromatherapy uses natural essential oils to improve the health of the mind, body, and spirit.

Aromatherapy has existed for thousands of years, most notably in the cultures of Egypt, China, and India. The ancients used natural resins, oils, and balms both medicinally and for religious purposes. Distillation of plant oils into essential oils did not happen until the 10th century in Persia. It wasn't until the 19th century that French physicians touted essential oils as possible cures for various diseases. The term aromatherapy was invented by a French perfumer and chemist Rene-Maurice in 1937, after discovering the healing properties of lavender oil on burns.

Today, essential oils and aromatherapy have become mainstream, with oils being available both online and even in common drugstores. However, essential oils are not regulated by the FDA, so you must choose your oils carefully and buy from a reputable producer such as Young Living or Plant Therapy. True essential oils do not contain any added synthetic fragrances, and if the bottle says the oil is flammable, it is not a true essential oil, as natural oils are not flammable.

Aromatherapy benefits

There are countless advantages to essential oils for health benefits. A few benefits include:

- Improves pain and inflammation (i.e., joint and muscle pain, arthritis, etc.)
- Improves sleep
- Heals skin (burns, cuts, scrapes, etc.)
- Reduces stress, anxiety, and depression
- Reduces headaches and migraines
- Alleviates nausea and improves digestion
- Boosts immunity by fighting viruses, bacteria, and fungi
- Helps relieve asthma, cold and flu symptoms by clearing congestion
- Fights fatigue

- Helps cancer patients with various symptoms
- Decreases symptoms of both menstruation and menopause

Aromatherapy and Reiki

Reiki practitioners use specific oils that align with the chakras (discussed in chapter two). Aromatherapy enhances the Reiki experience, creating a relaxing ambiance to help patients "go deeper" into their experience.

Some popular essential oils used in Reiki sessions include:

- Lavender and eucalyptus: Lavender and eucalyptus bring stress relief and deeper relaxation. Eucalyptus is also beneficial for the respiratory system, which is helpful during the deep breathing during Reiki sessions.
- Orange or peppermint: These invigorating scents are used at the end of

a session, to help slowly bring patients out of their deeply relaxed state.

●Vetiver: This oil is beneficial for more extreme cases of anxiety, such as anxiety disorder or the onset of a panic attack, as its earthy aroma can be grounding.

●Bergamot: Bergamot is a Meditteranean hybrid fruit that crosses oranges and lemons. This uplifting scent is used for chronic states of stress and anxiety, and the gentle scent is not overwhelming to most people.

●Frankincense: This bold, potent oil helps with many different physical ailments such as tension headaches, abdominal pain, and muscle soreness. It is also hailed as a potent antidepressant, with effects lasting for days after use.

If you are using oils for yourself, choose oils that appeal to you and don't cause reactions or headaches. If you are choosing oils for another person you are practicing on, talk to them first to see what scents appeal to them and what allergies or sensitivities they might have. Then you can decide on the appropriate oils to use in your session.

Essential oils can either be used diluted on the skin or diffused as a vapor in a diffuser. Note that the only oil can that be used undiluted on the skin is lavender. All other oils must be diluted in a carrier oil like jojoba or argan oil to prevent irritation. When using either method, be sure not to overload the senses with too much scent. Less is more with essential oils!

Conclusion

Achakra relates to the life-force power and transmits it; it is the equilibrium point within the body. Charka comes from the Sanskrit word, which describes a wheel or a sound energy sphere that is continuously spinning.

Some conventional Hindu scriptures say that a person's body has approximately 90,000 points of Chakra. However, seven Chakras are more critical than the rest. Such chakras live from the base of the spine to the top of the head.

The base or root chakras are the origins of these chakras. Then we move up the column with the Chakra of the sex or the navel, with the plexus of the stomach or the solar plexus, the Chakra of the heart, the Chakra of the throat, the Chakra of the brow or the third eye and the Chakra. Such seven significant chakras receive and transmit signals from the natural universe or the infinite cosmos. It affects an individual's religious, metaphysical, mental, cognitive, bodily, and psychological status.

Chakras have been defined in various ways, but they all have one common feature. Whether from Chinese medicine or the Hindu perspective, all these explanations are identical. It is the perception of people's experiences and the way that the human mind thinks and feels different emotions.

Whether we are awake or not, the chakras are in constant movement. The structure, behavior, physical conditions, glandular processes, and our thoughts and actions will affect this continuous activity. Nevertheless, if there is a chakra malfunction in one or more points that may be triggered by different reasons, a disequilibrium may evolve and become evident in other areas of our being.

It is believed that the chakras are associated with the endocrine joy in our bodies. If a chakra gets out of balance, then we can have so-called trouble in the normal behavior of the endocrine gland and everything connected or connected to that gland.

You can say that any significant illnesses or diseases that may affect your body can be associated with an unbalanced chakra. It is essential to maintain the correct balance of chakras to ensure that your body works correctly. While you may not see the physical characteristics of a disease or imbalance, you may see a difference in your emotions.

The repressed and overlooked emotional baggage we bear because of those traumatic experiences is one of the significant causes of a chakra imbalance. Most people usually enjoy their bad memories without realizing that these psychological toxins that are hidden inside them affect their cellular bodies.

Thus it is necessary once and for all to deal with emotional baggage to maintain a proper balance of the chakras, which initiates a healing process in order, to begin with, the physical self.

You should know that chakra healing is perfect for your body and that you can affect every one of your chakras directly. You can do so using methods such as Reiki treatment, color therapy, aromatherapy, pendulum chakra balance, crystals, or gemstones.

Many people like to do yoga classes that help with their breathing and physical exercises. Yoga is good to keep chakra balance in the body, as it allows people to concentrate.

Many approaches to treat chakras include meditation and guided visualization. This is often done through relaxing music CDs that help to promote natural healing by relaxing techniques. It helps reduce pressure and harness our mind's energy.

Even when we know that we can't touch or see our Chakra, we can help each other to make the best of our bodies.

The human body needs to be healthy and properly fed so that we can have a balanced chakra. Foods help to maintain the balance of each of the seven primary chakras.

Root vegetables and foods rich in protein and spices help feed the root chakra. The holy Chakra that blends sex and imagination is nurtured by things such as sweet fruit, nuts, cinnamon, coffee, and seeds such as sesame and cabbage. The solar plexus chakra feeds spicy mintstones, dairy products, yogurt, pasta, bread, and cereals that inspire our sense of self-reliance and self-love.

Are you aware that the heart chakra best works on leafy vegetables and even many green tea types? The Chakra of the throat always needs a lot of hydrating fluids.

Water and even fruit juices like apple and orange juice are the most active liquids.

The 3rd eye chakra thrives on strawberries, blueberries, and wine.

The crown chakra needs proper detoxification in our emotional and spiritual center. This is achieved by ceremonial inhalation of spices, fasts, and incense.

We are always safe by trying to keep our chakras balanced. It makes us more in tune with our surroundings and allows others to live in the spiritual world in which we live.

www.ingramcontent.com/pod-product-compliance
Lightning Source LLC
Chambersburg PA
CBHW072005070526
44583CB00015B/1345